BLUEPRINTS IN RADIOLOGY

high attenuation - white.

BLUEPRINTS in
RADIOLOGY

Ryan W. Davis, MD
Radiology Resident
Cedars-Sinai Medical Center
Los Angeles, California

Mitchell S. Komaiko, MD
Director, Radiology Residency Program
Cedars-Sinai Medical Center
Los Angeles, California

Faculty Advisor:
Barry D. Pressman, MD, FACR
Chairman, Department of Radiology
Cedars-Sinai Medical Center
Los Angeles, California

Blackwell
Publishing

First Indian Reprint 2003

Blackwell Publishing, Inc., 350 Main Street, Malden, Massachusetts 02148-5018, USA
Blackwell Science Ltd, Osney Mead, Oxford OX2 0EL, UK
Blackwell Science Asia Pty Ltd, 550 Swanston Street, Carlton, Victoria 3053, Australia
Blackwell Verlag GmbH, Kurfürstendamm 57, 10707 Berlin, Germany

ISBN: 0-632-04588-4

Library of Congress Cataloging-in-Publication Data

Davis, Ryan W.
    Blueprints in radiology / by Ryan W. Davis, Mitchell S. Komaiko, Barry
D. Pressman.
        p. ; cm. — (Blueprints USMLE Steps 2 & 3 review series)
Includes index.
    ISBN 0-632-04588-4 (pbk. : alk. paper)
    1. Radiography, Medical—Outlines, syllabi, etc. 2. Radiography,
Medical—Examinations, questions, etc.
    [DNLM: 1. Diagnostic Imaging—methods—Examination Questions. 2.
Radiography—methods—Examination Questions. WN 18.2 D264b 2002] I.
Komaiko, Mitchell S. II. Pressman, Barry D. III. Title. IV. Blueprints.
    RC78.17 D385 2002
    616.07'572'076—dc21
                                        2002006042

A catalogue record for this title is available from the British Library

Acquisitions: Beverly Copland
Development: Angela Gagliano
Production: Debra Lally
Cover design: Hannus Design
Typesetter: Techbooks in York, PA
Printed and bound in India by Replika Press Pvt. Ltd., Kundli 131 028

For further information on Blackwell Publishing, visit our website:
www.blackwellscience.com

Notice: The indications and dosages of all drugs in this book have been recommended in the medical literature and conform to the practices of the general community. The medications described do not necessarily have specific approval by the Food and Drug Administration for use in the diseases and dosages for which they are recommended. The package insert for each drug should be consulted for use and dosage as approved by the FDA. Because standards for usage change, it is advisable to keep abreast of revised recommendations, particularly those concerning new drugs.

Contents

	Reviewers	vii
	Preface	ix
	Acknowledgments	xi
	Abbreviations	xiii
1	General Principles in Radiology	1
2	Head and Neck Imaging	8
3	Neurologic Imaging	22
4	Thoracic Imaging	31
5	Abdominal Imaging	55
6	Urologic Imaging	70
7	Obstetric and Gynecologic Imaging	76
8	Musculoskeletal Imaging	83
9	Pediatric Imaging	98
	Questions	111
	Answers	117
	Index	121

Reviewers

Michael W. Lamb, MD
PGY-1
Barnes-Jewish Hospital
Saint Louis, Missouri

Heather N. Malm
Des Moines University
Class of 2002
Des Moines, Iowa

George N. Scarlatis, MD
PGY-1
Evanston Northwestern Healthcare
Evanston, Illinois

Joshua D. Valtos
Emory University
Class of 2002
Atlanta, Georgia

Preface

Blueprints in Radiology continues the Blueprints series with concise chapters covering the most important topics needed to excel on the USMLE Step 2 & 3 exams and during internship.

This book was developed to provide a much-needed resource for medical students and interns on the fundamentals of Radiology. It is not meant to be comprehensive, but rather, a concise review for board exams and medical school rotations. Chapters are divided by organ system and explain the most common imaging studies for each system. Each chapter includes classic case presentations and associated images that are likely to appear on the board exams. You can then test yourself with Q&A's at the end of the book.

We hope that you find *Blueprints in Radiology* to be both valuable and beneficial in your studies of Radiology. We welcome your comments and feedback to blue@blacksci.com.

Ryan W. Davis, MD
Mitchell S. Komaiko, MD

Acknowledgments

I would like to thank Dr. Mitchell S. Komaiko and Dr. Barry D. Pressman for their time, effort, and support in this project. I would also like to thank Michael Catron and the residents of Cedars-Sinai imaging for their encouragement. A special thanks goes to Dr. Carl Fuhrman whose wonderful teaching led me to a career in radiology.

This book is dedicated to my parents, and all parents like them, who deferred many dreams so that their children could reach for theirs.

RD

Abbreviations

ACA	anterior cerebral artery
AP	anterior-posterior
ARDS	aquired respiratory distress syndrome
CA	carcinoma
CBC	complete blood count
CN	cranial nerve
COPD	chronic obstructive pulmonary disease
CT	computed tomography
CXR	chest x-ray; chest radiograph
DIP	distal inter-phalangeal joint
DISIDA	diisopropyl iminodiacetic acid; diisofenin
DTPA	diethylene triamine penta-acetic acid
EEC	endometrial echo complex
ESR	erythrocyte sedimentation rate
GCS	Glasgow coma score
GI	gastrointestinal
GSW	gunshot wound
HIDA	dimethyl iminodiacetic acid
HIV	human immunodeficiency virus
HLA	human leukocyte antigen
HU	Hounsfield Units
IAC	internal auditory canal
IV	intravenous
IVC	inferior vena cava

IVP	intravenous pyelogram
KUB	kidneys, ureters, bladder radiograph
LAT	lateral
MAG-3	methyl-acetyl-glycine-glycine-glycine
MCA	middle cerebral artery
MCP	meta-carpal phalangeal
MHz	Megahertz
MMSE	mini-mental status exam
MRA	magnetic resonance angiography
MRI	magnetic resonance imaging
MVA	motor vehicle accident
NF	neurofibromatosis
PA	posterior-anterior
PCA	posterior cerebral artery
PET	positron emission tomography
PIP	proximal interphalangeal joint
PMN	polymorphonuclear cells
RDS	respiratory distress syndrome (newborn)
RF	radiofrequency, also rheumatoid factor
SGOT	serum glutamic-oxaloacetic transaminase; AST
SVC	superior vena cava
TB	tuberculosis
UPJ	uretero-pelvic junction
US	Ultrasound
UVJ	uretero-vesicular junction
V/Q	ventilation-perfusion
WBC	white blood cell

General Principles in Radiology

INTRODUCTION

In 1895, Dutch physicist Wilhelm Roentgen discovered the x-ray, and since that time, many uses for it have been developed in both diagnostic and therapeutic medicine. The specialty of radiology includes conventional techniques that use ionizing radiation: radiography (plain film); fluoroscopy; computed tomography (CT); and nuclear medicine. It also includes the techniques of magnetic resonance imaging (MRI) and ultrasound, which produce images with magnetic fields and sound waves respectively, thereby avoiding the risks of radiation.

RADIOGRAPHY AND FLUOROSCOPY

A standard x-ray machine (Figure 1-1) generates high-energy photons, or x-rays as they are also called, with a high-voltage electric current. The x-rays are directed in a focused beam towards the patient. They will either pass through the patient to the film; be absorbed by the patient's tissues; or scatter and not provide diagnostic information. As the x-rays reach the cassette and interact with the radiographic film, their energy is converted into visible light, which exposes the film, and creates the familiar radiograph. In fluoroscopy, the film is replaced by the image intensifier, which allows a digital image to be seen on a television monitor in real time.

The radiograph itself is a two-dimensional representation of the three-dimensional structures of the patient's body. These structures are visible because of the differences in attenuation of the x-ray beam. Attenuation refers to the process by which x-rays are removed

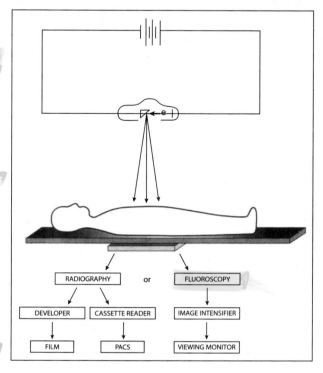

Figure 1-1. Plain film radiography and fluoroscopy. (Illustration by Shawn Girsberger Graphic Design.)

TABLE 1-1

The Five Main Radiodensities on a Standard Radiograph.
(Table Rendered by Shawn Girsberger Graphic Design)

Material	Effective Atomic Number	Density (g/cm³)	Color on Film
Air	7.6	RADIOLUCENT 0.001	
Fat	5.9	0.9	
Water (Organ tissue, muscle skin, blood	7.4	1	
Bone	14.0	2	
Metal	82.0	RADIODENSE 11	

from the primary x-ray beam through absorption and scatter. Attenuated x-rays are essentially "blocked" and never reach the film to expose it. The degree of attenuation by the tissues of the body is based on three main factors: the tissue thickness in the line of the x-ray beam; the density of the tissue; and the atomic number of the material through which the beam passes (Table 1-1).

Unexposed film, which corresponds to high attenuation of the x-ray beam, appears bright on the radiograph, as with bone, for example. Exposed film, which corresponds to low attenuation of the x-ray beam, appears dark, as with the air of the lungs. The terms radiolucency and radiodensity relate to attenuation along the same scale in that air is the most radiolucent and bone is the most radiodense. A gradient of gray, corresponding to all the remaining tissue types, lies between these two extremes. Four main tissue types are distinguished on a radiograph, and, in order of increasing attenuation, they are air, fat, soft tissue, and bone.

Distinctions between tissues can only be made when there is an interface with differences in density between the tissues. For instance, air bronchograms are evident in a lung segment with pneumonia because there is an interface between the air inside the bronchi and the pus-filled alveoli of the lung tissue. As a demonstration, a balloon filled with water is placed inside of a glass, also filled with water (Figures 1-2a, 1-2b). Because there is essentially a "water-water" interface, with the thin membrane of the balloon

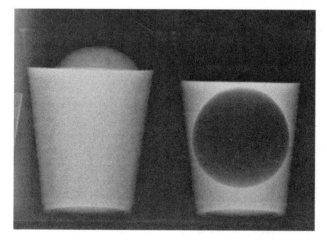

Figure 1-2a. Radiographic demonstration of interfaces. On the left, a balloon filled with water rests inside a cup filled with water. The "water-water" interface cannot be seen because there is no difference in attenuation. On the right, a balloon filled with air rests inside a cup filled with water. An "air-water" interface is demonstrated and the air appears black inside the water, which is white. (Used with permission of Cedars-Sinai Medical Center, Los Angeles, California.)

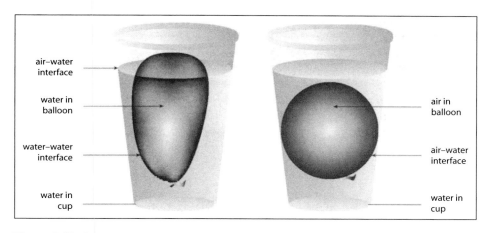

Figure 1-2b. Diagrammatic representation of the radiographic interfaces in Figure 1-2a. (Illustration by Shawn Girsberger Graphic Design.)

between, the balloon is not seen on a radiograph. Fill the balloon with air, creating an "air-water" interface, and the shape of the balloon becomes evident on the radiograph.

Plain radiographs are useful as first-line examinations of the chest, abdomen, and skeletal structures. Some common indications for chest radiographs are shortness of breath, chest pain, and cough. For abdominal plain films, common indications are abdominal pain, vomiting, and trauma. Skeletal films are useful in the evaluation of osseous trauma, arthritis, bone neoplasms, metabolic bone disease, and congenital dysplasias.

◆ KEY POINTS ◆

1. The familiar radiograph is a two-dimensional representation of the three-dimensional structures of the patient's body.

2. Four main tissue types are distinguished on a radiograph, and, in order of increasing attenuation, they are air, fat, soft tissue, and bone.

3. Distinctions between tissues can only be made when there is an interface with differences in density between the tissues.

4. Plain radiographs are useful as first-line examinations of the chest, abdomen, and skeletal structures.

CT

CT is a method of using x-rays in multiple projections to produce axial images of the body. The image production differs from conventional radiography in that the x-rays pass through the patient to highly sensitive detectors instead of film. These detectors then send the information to a computer that reconstructs the images (Figure 1-3). The images are displayed in anatomic position as if one is observing the patient while standing at the feet, looking towards the head. Any body part can be imaged, but generally, exams are divided into head, neck, spine, chest, abdomen, pelvis, and extremities. The patient lies supine on the exam table, which moves horizontally through the frame or gantry, as it is commonly called.

In CT, adjacent anatomic structures are delineated by differences in attenuation between them. Again, attenuation refers to the physical properties of the molecules in the body, which contribute to absorption and scatter of the x-ray beams. These properties differentially prevent some of the x-rays from reaching the detectors on the opposite side of the gantry.

CT is more sensitive than conventional plain film in distinguishing differences of tissue density, which are displayed in Hounsfield units (HU), in a range of approximately (-1000) to $(+1000)$ corresponding to a gradient scale of gray. Generally, one can divide densities for CT into seven general categories (with their HU ranges):

TABLE 1-2

Hounsfield Units on CT. (Table Rendered by Shawn Girsberger Graphic Design)

CT into seven general categories (with their HU ranges):

1. Air (−1000 to −200 HU)
2. Fat (−50 to 0 HU)
3. Water (0 to 10 HU)
4. Soft tissue (20 to 50 HU)
5. Non-flowing blood (50 to 70 HU)
6. Bone (+300 to −500 HU)
7. Metal (+500 to +1000 HU)

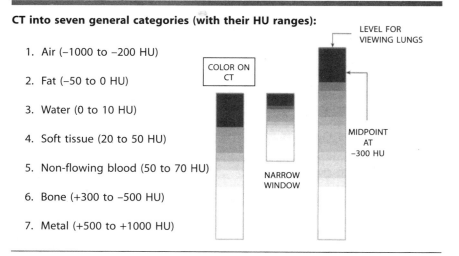

Two important concepts arise in discussion of the Hounsfield unit grayscale; the concepts of "window" and "level." Window refers to the range across which the computer will display the shades of gray on the monitor for viewing. A narrow window produces greater contrast. Level is the midpoint value in Hounsfield units of the scale and is used to preferentially view different types of tissue. For example, to examine lung detail, one would preferentially choose a low value (−300 HU) for the level, instead of the higher HU values of soft tissue and bone.

Common uses of CT include any part of the body where fine anatomic detail or subtle distinction between tissue types is necessary for diagnosis. Examples include a head CT to exclude bleeding or skull fracture in head trauma; a chest CT to evaluate nodules or masses; an abdominal CT for metastatic workup or in fever of unknown origin to exclude abscess; and a skeletal CT to evaluate subtle fractures not clearly seen on plain films.

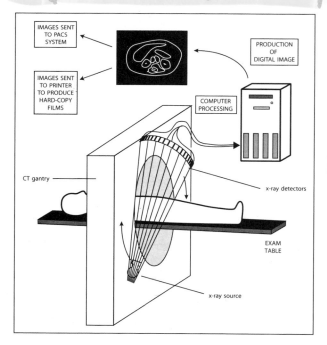

Figure 1-3. Standard computed tomography (CT) system and production of axial CT images. (Illustration by Shawn Girsberger Graphic Design.)

◆ **KEY POINTS** ◆

1. CT is a method of using x-rays to produce axial images of the body, which are viewed as if looking from the feet up towards the head.
2. CT is more sensitive than conventional plain film in distinguishing differences of tissue density.
3. Common uses of CT include any part of the body where fine anatomic detail or subtle distinction between tissue types is necessary for diagnosis.

NUCLEAR MEDICINE

Nuclear medicine differs from conventional radiography in several fundamental ways. First, rather than delivering x-rays externally through the patient to produce an image, a dose of radiation is given <u>internally</u> to the patient and the x-rays are counted as they leave his or her body. Second, some nuclear medicine studies provide functional information in addition to the anatomic information of conventional radiographic techniques. The radiation dose or radionuclide is usually given either orally or intravenously and has an affinity for certain organs. As the radionuclide decays, it emits gamma radiation, which is detected by special cameras that count the number of emitted photons and send the information to a computer (Figure 1-4). The computer processes the data with regard to the source location and number of counts to form an image or series of images over time.

Common uses of nuclear medicine studies are: ventilation-perfusion (V/Q) scan for suspected pulmonary embolism; di-isopropyl iminodiacetic acid (DISIDA) scan for suspected acute cholecystitis; bone scan or positron emission tomography (PET) for metastatic work-up; diethylene triamene penta-acetic acid (DTPA) renal scan for renal failure; Gallium scan for lymphoma or occult infection; Indium tagged white blood cell scan for occult infection; iodine-123 scan for thyroid nodules; technetium tagged red blood cell scan for gastrointestinal bleeding and hepatic hemangioma evaluation.

◆ KEY POINTS ◆

1. In nuclear medicine studies, a dose of radiation is given internally to the patient and the x-rays are counted as they leave his or her body.

2. Some nuclear medicine studies provide functional information in addition to the anatomic information of conventional radiographic techniques.

ULTRASOUND

In ultrasonography (US), a probe is applied to the patient's skin, and a high frequency (1 to 20 MHz) beam of sound waves is focused on the area of interest (Figure 1-5). The

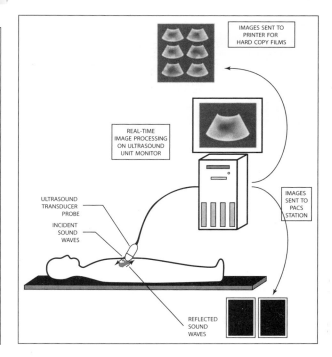

Figure 1-4. Standard two-head gamma camera and production of nuclear medicine scintigraphy images. (Illustration by Shawn Girsberger Graphic Design.)

Figure 1-5. Standard ultrasound system and production of ultrasonographic images. (Illustration by Shawn Girsberger Graphic Design.)

sound waves propagate through different tissues at different velocities, with denser tissues allowing the sound waves to move faster. A detector measures the time it takes for the wave to reflect and return to the probe. Tissue density is determined by the reflection time and an image is produced on the screen for the ultrasonographer to see in real time. Normal soft tissue appears as medium echogenicity, the term for brightness on ultrasound. Fat is usually more echogenic than soft tissue. Simple fluid, such as bile, has low echogenicity, appears dark, and often has "through-transmission" or brightness beyond it. Complex fluid, such as blood or pus, may have strands or septations within it, and generally has lower through-transmission than simple fluid. Calcification usually appears as high echogenicity with posterior "shadowing," or a "dark band" beyond it. Air does not transmit sound waves well and does not permit imaging beyond it, as the sound waves do not reflect back to the transducer. Therefore, bowel gas and lung tissue are a hindrance to ultrasound imaging.

Common uses of ultrasound include evaluating the gall bladder for suspected cholecystitis, the pancreas for pancreatitis, and the right lower quadrant of the abdomen in suspected appendicitis. Other indications include evaluation of the liver, pancreas or kidneys for masses or evidence of obstruction. Ultrasound is also very helpful in the evaluation of pelvic pain in women and in suspected ectopic pregnancy, ovarian torsion, or pelvic masses. Finally, with the use of Doppler imaging in US, which detects flow velocity and direction, one can image blood vessels such as the aorta for suspected aneurysm, and the deep leg veins or portal vein for thrombosis.

◆ KEY POINTS ◆

1. Ultrasound imaging uses the reflection of high-frequency sound waves to generate images of the patient's internal organs.

2. Bowel gas and lung tissue are a hindrance to ultrasound imaging.

3. Common uses of ultrasound include evaluating the gall bladder, pancreas, liver, and kidneys for various pathologic conditions. Ultrasound is also useful in the assessment of acute pelvic pain in women and various other pathologic conditions of the pelvic organs.

MRI

In general terms, MRI utilizes the physical principle that hydrogen protons will align when placed within a strong magnetic field. To obtain an MRI scan, the patient lies on the table within the scanner tube and is surrounded by a high-intensity magnetic field (Figure 1-6). Protons in the patient's tissues align with the vector of the magnetic field and a radiofrequency (RF) pulse is emitted from the transmitter coils, causing the protons to "deflect" perpendicular to their original vector. When the RF pulse ceases, the protons "relax" back to their original position, releasing energy, which is detected by the receiver coils of the scanner. The patient's tissues will generate different signals depending on relative hydrogen proton composition. These signals are processed by a computer to produce the final image.

There are several advantages of MRI over CT. First, MRI does not use ionizing radiation, and therefore avoids its potential harmful effects. Second, images can be easily obtained in any plane, rather than only the

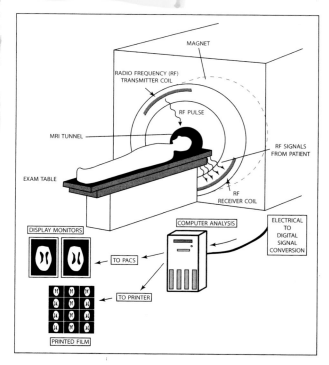

Figure 1-6. Standard magnetic resonance imaging (MRI) magnet and production of MR images. (Illustration by Shawn Girsberger Graphic Design.)

transverse plane as with CT. Finally, MRI generally provides better anatomic detail of soft tissues, and is better at detecting subtle pathologic differences. The disadvantages are that MRI takes much longer to scan a patient than CT, is more expensive, and has more contraindications such as pacemakers, aneurysm clips, and metallic foreign bodies, all of which may be adversely affected by the magnetic field.

◆ KEY POINTS ◆

1. MRI utilizes the physical principle that hydrogen protons will align when placed within a strong magnetic field.
2. The patient's tissues will generate different signals for the final MR image, depending on relative hydrogen proton composition.
3. MRI does not use ionizing radiation.
4. MRI generally provides better anatomic detail of soft tissues than CT.

CONTRAST MATERIAL

Contrast material increases the differences in density between anatomic structures. Gastrointestinal contrast agents such as barium and gastrograffin are used to outline the entire gastrointestinal tract for CT and fluoroscopic exams. Intravenous contrast agents such as iodine-based contrast for CT and gadolinium for MRI are used to visualize vascular structures and provide enhancement of organs.

Intravenous iodine-based contrast is seen within blood vessels, allowing them to be distinguished from lymph nodes and other soft tissue structures of similar anatomic dimensions. It is therefore preferentially seen in areas of relatively high blood flow, identifying tumors, abscesses, or areas of inflammation. Contrast passes through leaky vascular spaces in tumors, increasing the attenuation of the tissue and making it more conspicuous. Iodine-based contrast also frequently yields a diagnosis based on its absence. For example, a filling defect within a blood vessel or solid organ likely indicates thrombus, hypoperfusion or infarct.

Intravenous iodine-based contrast is mandatory for a chest CT if pulmonary embolism is suspected. Other uses include suspected solid organ tumor to look for enhancement. If an abscess is suspected, contrast is helpful to delineate the margins of an infected cavity, due to the relative hyperemia in the abscess walls, which appear as high attenuation on a CT scan.

The risks and benefits of intravenous iodine-based contrast should be considered before using it for a patient who has any renal compromise due to the risk of causing acute renal failure. IV iodine-based contrast is usually not given if the patient's creatinine is above 1.5, unless the study is absolutely necessary. One example of this would be in a case of trauma with suspected vascular, renal or ureteral injury. The contrast also carries a risk of causing allergic reactions, including anaphylaxis; however allergic reactions are significantly less common with the newer non-ionic contrast agents. Patients with a history of clinically significant allergic reaction to iodine should still be premedicated with diphenhydramine hydrochloride and an H2-blocker such as cimetidine or ranitidine. If intravenous iodine contrast is to be given to a patient who uses the antidiabetic medication metformin, the medication must not be given for the following 48 hours due to the risk of metabolic acidosis.

◆ KEY POINTS ◆

1. Contrast material increases the differences in density between anatomic structures.
2. Intravenous iodine-based contrast carries the risks of causing acute renal failure and allergic reactions.

2 Head and Neck Imaging

TRAUMA-FACIAL BONE FRACTURES

Anatomy

The facial bones and paranasal sinuses provide a natural "shock absorber," which, in addition to the calvarium, protect the brain during head trauma. The most commonly fractured skull bones are the nasal bones, maxillary antrum, the walls of the orbit, and the zygomatic arch (Figure 2-1).

Etiology

There are two major categories of facial trauma: blunt and penetrating injuries. The most common causes of blunt trauma are motor vehicle accidents, falls, and assaults. Gunshot wounds are the most common penetrating traumas.

Epidemiology

Motor vehicle accidents are the most common cause of facial trauma in young adults. In the elderly, ground-level falls are the most common cause. Elderly patients are unable to extend their arms to break the fall. Often, patients in the hospital try to get out of bed in the middle of the night, become disoriented in the unfamiliar setting of their hospital room, and subsequently fall. Syncope, orthostatic hypotension, and weakness from prolonged bedrest place these patients at increased risk for a fall.

History

In motor vehicle accidents, occult injuries occur more frequently in unrestrained passengers, so it is important to determine if a patient was restrained or unrestrained. If the trauma occurred more than 24 hours prior to presentation, then questions regarding headaches, visual changes, and sinus drainage become important as these symptoms may represent stable but significant facial trauma. Sinus drainage may be an indication of cerebrospinal fluid leakage from an open frontal or sphenoid sinus fracture. Open sinus fractures are extremely important to detect as they may lead to secondary intracerebral infections such as meningitis or abscess.

Physical Examination

Ecchymoses, soft tissue swelling, and hematomas are the most common physical findings in facial trauma. Decreased visual acuity or strabismus are often present with orbital fractures and associated intraocular muscle or cranial nerve injury.

Diagnostic Evaluation

In acute trauma, the overall evaluation begins with an assessment of the patient's stability. Once airway, breathing, and circulation are established, and a focused physical exam is performed, the radiographic evaluation can begin. This evaluation may, on rare occasion, begin with plain films in uncomplicated cases; however, a non-contrast CT scan of the head is usually done to exclude intracranial injury in addition to facial fractures in a single exam. A head CT is especially important in patients with neurologic changes and/or decreased score on the Glasgow coma score (GCS) or mini-mental status exam (MMSE). These alterations in mental status may indicate intracranial injury that CT will detect, but plain films will not.

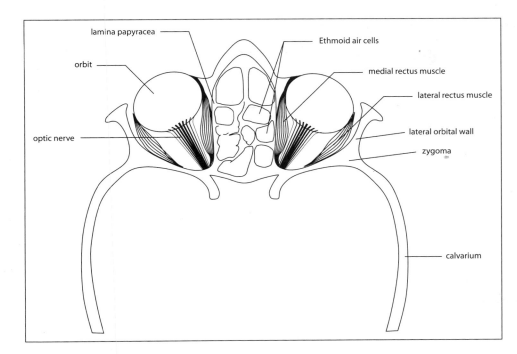

lamina papyracea
Ethmoid air cells
orbit
medial rectus muscle
lateral rectus muscle
lateral orbital wall
optic nerve
zygoma
calvarium

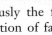

Figure 2-1. Anatomy of facial bones at the level of the orbits. (Illustration by Shawn Girsberger Graphic Design.)

Radiologic Findings

Areas of importance on plain films are the orbits and the maxillary sinuses. "Blowout fractures" of the orbital floor are noted as a discontinuity of the bone cortex projecting into the ipsilateral maxillary sinus, best seen on a Caldwell view plain film or a coronal view CT scan. An air-fluid level in the maxillary sinus is an associated finding in some cases and represents blood within the sinus. A soft tissue mass projecting from the orbit into the maxillary sinus suggests herniation of orbital soft tissues.

Essential areas to evaluate on the head CT are the calvarium, orbital walls, paranasal sinuses, and mastoid air cells. Inspection of the calvarium includes bone and soft tissue windows to look for fractures, soft tissue swelling, and hematomas that indicate areas of direct trauma. Subtle fractures are commonly found in the bone adjacent to areas of soft tissue swelling. Assessment of the orbits by CT includes axial and coronal views with bone and soft tissue windows. Coronal views are important to exclude orbital floor fractures, and soft tissue windowing is crucial to exclude muscle entrapment or optic nerve impingement (Figures 2-2, 2-3). In the paranasal sinuses, air-fluid levels of high attenuation represent acute blood (Figure 2-4), likely associated with subtle fractures. Fluid in the mastoid air cells is always pathologic; in the setting of trauma, it likely represents blood, with an associated skull-base fracture (Figure 2-5).

◆ KEY POINTS ◆

1. Plain radiographs were previously the first step in the radiographic evaluation of facial trauma; however, a non-contrast CT scan of the head may preferentially be done to exclude facial fractures and intracranial injury in a single exam, especially in patients with mental status changes.

2. Air-fluid levels in the sinuses in the setting of trauma likely represent blood and indicate an occult fracture.

3. With orbital fractures, CT with bone and soft tissue windows should be used to exclude muscle entrapment or optic nerve impingement.

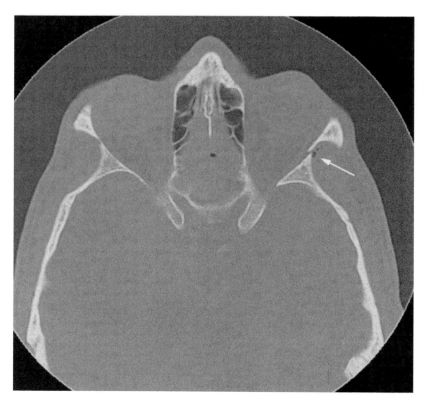

Figure 2-2. Fracture of the left lateral orbital wall on CT with bone windows. (Used with permission of Cedars-Sinai Medical Center, Los Angeles, California.)

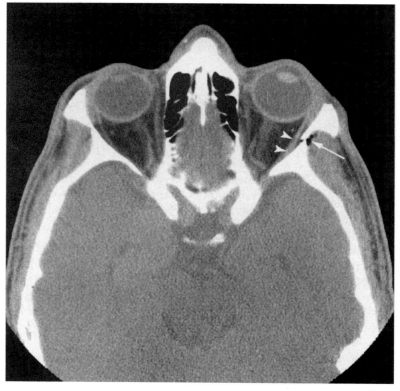

Figure 2-3. Fracture of the left lateral orbital wall on CT with soft tissue windows. There is close approximation of the fracture fragments to the lateral rectus muscle. In this case, there was no muscle entrapment. (Used with permission of Cedars-Sinai Medical Center, Los Angeles, California.)

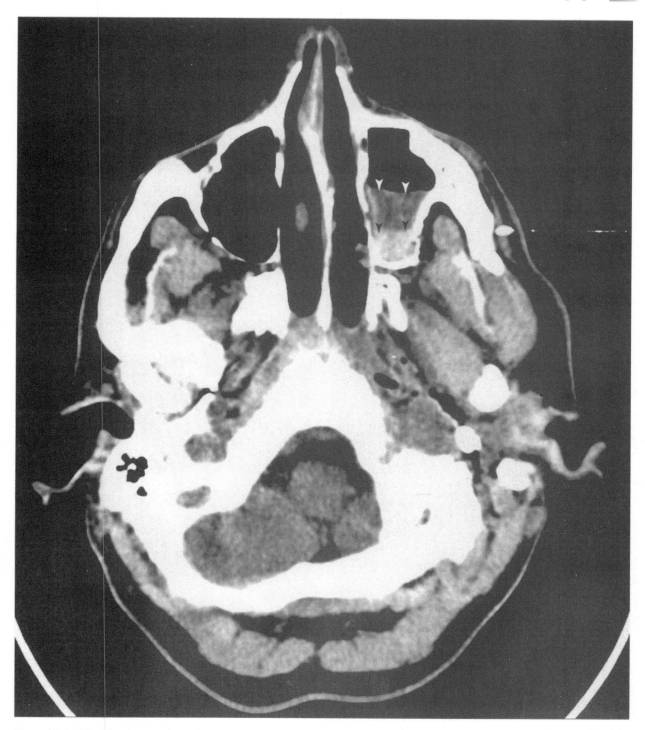

Figure 2-4. CT of the head at the level of the maxillary sinuses reveals an air-fluid level in the left maxillary sinus. The fluid has two different densities, with higher density fluid layering dependently. This represents blood separated into plasma on top and red cells on the bottom. (Used with permission of Cedars-Sinai Medical Center, Los Angeles, California.)

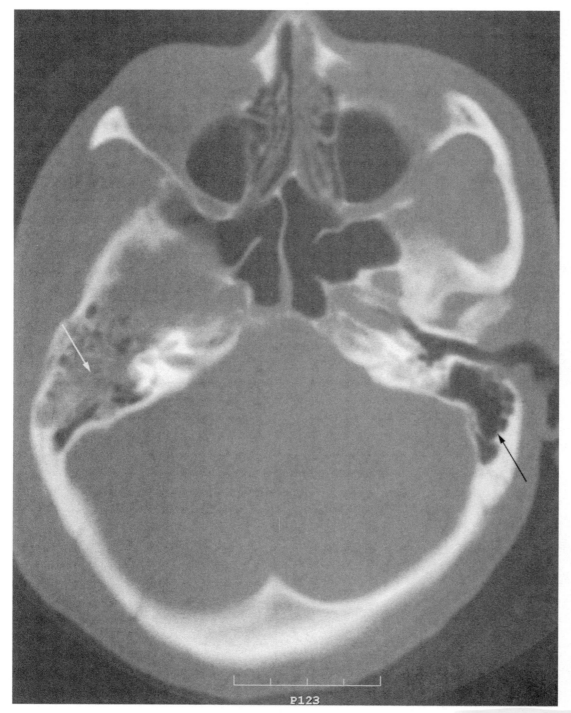

Figure 2-5. CT of the head at the level of the skull base with bone windowing, demonstrating fluid in the patient's right mastoid air cells (white arrow) compared to the normal left side (black arrow). The patient had an occult skull-base fracture. (Used with permission of Cedars-Sinai Medical Center, Los Angeles, California.)

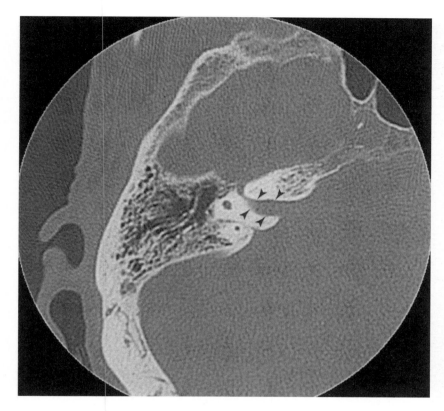

Figure 2-6. CT of the head showing a normal right internal auditory canal. (Used with permission of Cedars-Sinai Medical Center, Los Angeles, California.)

ACOUSTIC SCHWANNOMA/ VESTIBULOCOCHLEAR SCHWANNOMA

Anatomy

Cranial nerves VII and VIII run in the internal auditory canal (IAC), which angles horizontally from the cerebellopontine angle toward the petrous bone of the skull base. The open canal can usually be seen on at least one slice of a standard axial head CT (Figure 2-6). MRI is needed for fine detail of the nerves themselves (Figure 2-7).

Etiology

Acoustic schwannomas, also known as vestibulo-cochlear schwannomas or acoustic neuromas, arise from the Schwann cells of the axonal myelin sheaths. Schwannomas make up approximately 8% of all intracranial neoplasms and fall under the more general group of nerve sheath tumors, which also includes neurofibromas and malignant nerve sheath tumors.

Epidemiology

Most acoustic schwannomas occur de novo, however neurofibromatosis (NF) is the condition most commonly associated with them. NF type I (NF-I) represents 95% of the cases of neurofibromatosis and has an incidence of 1 in 2500 births. NF type II (NF-II) has an incidence of 1 in 50,000 and represents 5% of neurofibromatosis cases. However, if there are bilateral vestibular schwannomas, this is essentially pathognomonic for NF-II.

History

Patients complain of gradual onset hearing loss, which may be unilateral or bilateral. Depending on the extent of the schwannoma, there may be vertigo, tinnitus, or an internal ear infection.

Physical Examination

Visual inspection of the external ear canal and tympanic membrane should be performed. Hearing and vibratory sensation can be tested with the Rinne and Weber tests using tuning forks of different frequencies. The eyes

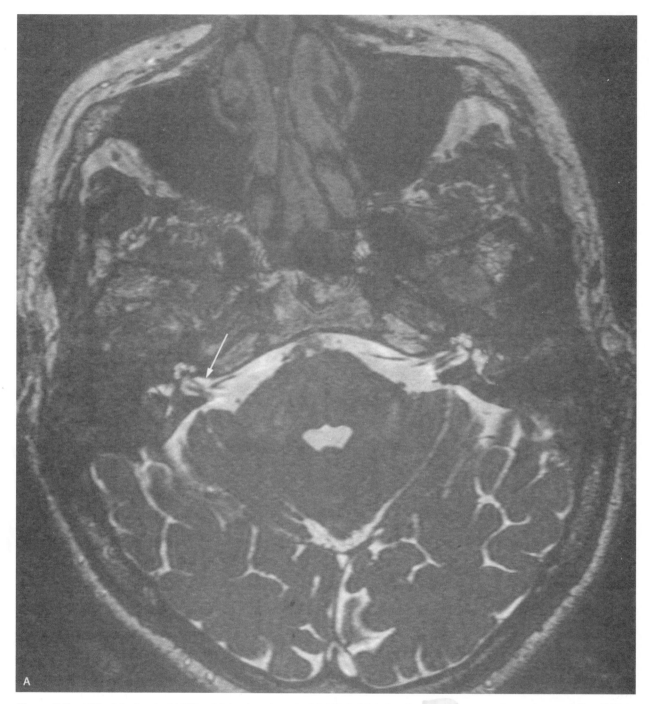

Figure 2-7a. MRI of the head with T2-weighting (cerebrospinal fluid is bright) showing normal course of cranial nerves VII and VIII into the internal auditory canals. (Used with permission of Cedars-Sinai Medical Center, Los Angeles, California.)

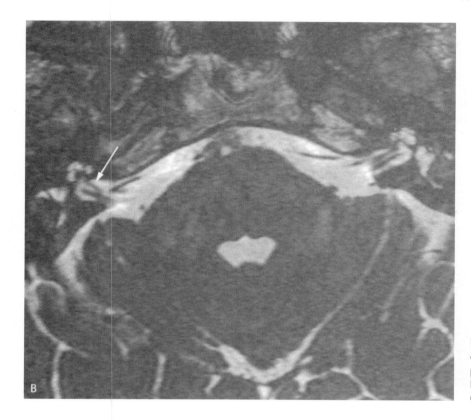

Figure 2-7b. Magnification view of Figure 2-7a. (Used with permission of Cedars-Sinai Medical Center, Los Angeles, California.)

should be tested for nystagmus and with an ophthalmoscope for papilledema from hydrocephalus caused by obstruction of the normal flow of cerebrospinal fluid.

Diagnostic Evaluation

Contrast-enhanced CT scan of the head is an appropriate screening examination for suspected acoustic schwannoma. Osseous erosion is important for detecting acoustic schwannoma on CT. MRI with gadolinium contrast is the imaging modality of choice. Thin sections (3mm) through the temporal bone on CT or basal cisterns on MRI may be required for diagnosis.

Radiologic Findings

A brightly enhancing mass in the IAC or within the cerebellopontine angle is the most common finding of acoustic schwannoma, and may be seen on either CT or MRI. A vestibular schwannoma may be difficult to distinguish from a meningioma, which classically has a broad dural tail that the schwannoma does not. A meningioma forms a broad base with the adjacent bone, while the schwannoma does not. Acoustic schwannoma extends along the course of the seventh and eighth nerves, often into the IAC (Figure 2-8). The IAC will likely be enlarged due to gradual expansion of the tumor (Figure 2-9) which is best seen on CT with bone windowing.

◆ KEY POINTS ◆

1. Acoustic neuroma, more properly called a vestibular schwannoma, arises from Schwann cells, which comprise the myelin sheaths of axons.

2. Nearly all patients with bilateral acoustic schwannomas have Neurofibromatosis type II.

3. Patients with acoustic schwannomas complain of gradual onset hearing loss.

4. An enhancing mass in the internal auditory canal or within the cerebellopontine angle, on either CT or MRI, is the most common finding of vestibular schwannoma.

5. MRI is the imaging modality of choice.

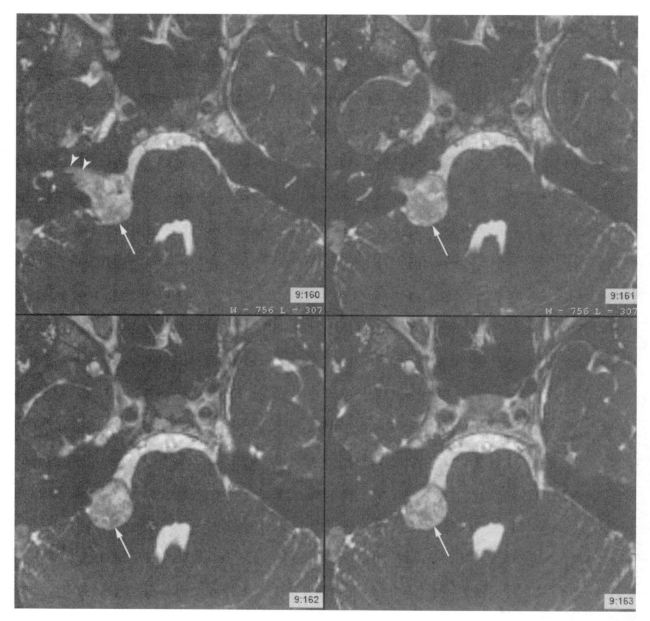

Figure 2-8. Acoustic schwannoma in the right cerebellopontine angle on T2-weighted MRI. (Used with permission of Cedars-Sinai Medical Center, Los Angeles, California.)

NF-I often has associated findings of optic gliomas, cerebral astrocytomas, scoliosis, and intraspinal neurofibromas. NF-II commonly has associated findings of multiple meningiomas and spinal nerve schwannomas.

HEAD AND NECK CANCER

Anatomy

Mass lesions of the head and neck may be difficult to classify based on radiologic appearance alone, but the

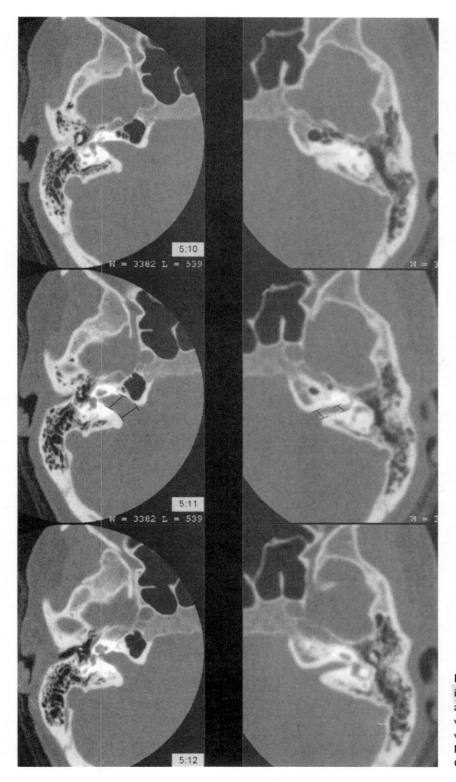

Figure 2-9. Expansion of right internal auditory canal by acoustic schwannoma on CT with bone windowing. (Used with permission of Cedars-Sinai Medical Center, Los Angeles, California.)

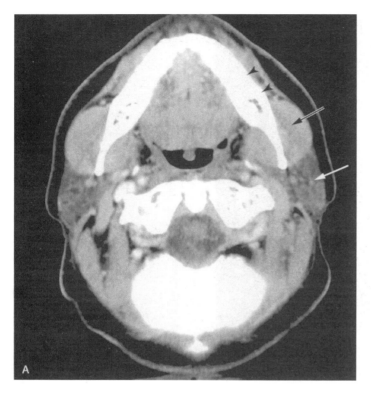

A

Figure 2-10a. Normal CT of the head with soft-tissue windowing at the level of the parotid glands (arrow). (Used with permission of Cedars-Sinai Medical Center, Los Angeles, California.)

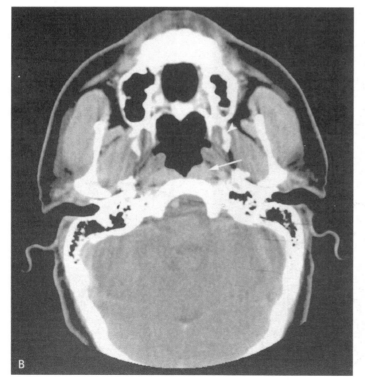

B

Figure 2-10b. Normal CT of the head at the level of the pterygoid plates (arrowhead) and nasopharyngeal soft tissues (white arrow). (Used with permission of Cedars-Sinai Medical Center, Los Angeles, California.)

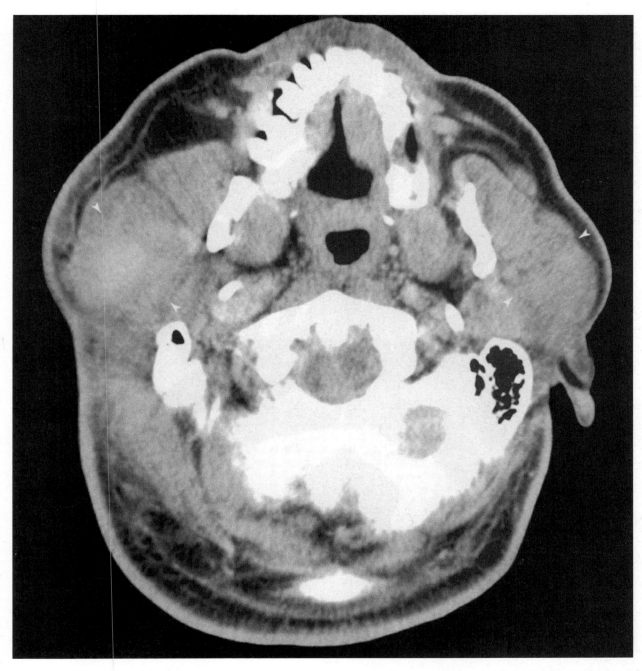

Figure 2-11. Parotid carcinoma. Bilateral parotid masses (between arrowheads) seen on contrast-enhanced CT scan of the neck. There are areas of necrosis suggesting rapid growth of the tumor, which has outgrown its blood supply. (Used with permission of Cedars-Sinai Medical Center, Los Angeles, California.)

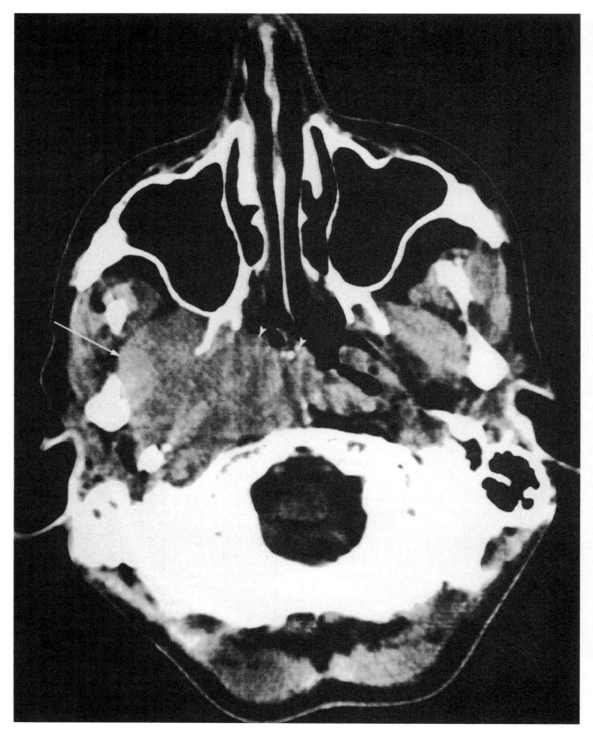

Figure 2-12. Pterygopalatine fossa carcinoma. CT scan of the neck demonstrates a large right pterygopalatine fossa mass. (Used with permission of Cedars-Sinai Medical Center, Los Angeles, California.)

differential diagnosis can be narrowed by identifying the adjacent anatomic structures and determining the most likely tissue type of origin. The most common sites of head and neck cancer are the vocal cords, the pterygopalatine fossa, the cavernous sinus, and the nasopharyngeal soft tissues (Figure 2-10).

Etiology

There are three basic tissue types that give rise to the majority of head and neck malignancies: squamous epithelium, lymphoid tissue, and salivary glands. Squamous cell carcinoma is by far the most common type of head and neck cancer. The salivary glands may also have tumors that are specific to each gland. For example, the parotid gland commonly has benign tumors (80%) such as pleomorphic adenomas and Warthin's tumors. The parotid gland also has malignant tumors (20%) such as adenocarcinoma, adenocystic carcinoma, squamous cell carcinoma, and mucoepidermoid carcinoma. Thyroid neoplasms may be benign such as thyroid adenoma, or malignant such as follicular, papillary, and anaplastic carcinoma.

Epidemiology

Head and neck cancers generally occur in the fourth to eighth decades. Risk factors include smoking and oral tobacco use. There is an increased risk of thyroid cancer with prior radiation exposure.

History

Symptoms depend on the location, the origin, and the type of tumor. Patients with squamous cell carcinoma of the pharynx complain of nasal obstruction, epistaxis, facial pain, or headache. Tumors of the larynx often cause hoarseness, changes in voice tone, or dysphagia. Lymphoma frequently presents with constitutional symptoms such as fever, fatigue, and weight loss, in addition to cervical lymph node enlargement.

Physical Exam

Examination of the throat commonly reveals a mass arising from the palate, or within the nasopharynx. Palpation of enlarged cervical lymph nodes is frequent.

Radiologic Findings

Both CT and MRI may be used for examination of the head and neck. MRI has the advantage of excellent soft tissue contrast and demonstration of the extent of a soft tissue mass. CT has the advantage of detecting involvement of osseous structures with osseous erosion or abnormalities of the paranasal sinuses.

Disruption of normal anatomic spaces and vascular relationships is a useful finding when surveying the extent of a tumor, and may give clues as to its origin. For example, a tumor of the parotid gland may push the carotid artery posteriorly and/or medially (Figure 2-11). A tumor of the pterygopalatine fossa may be seen on physical exam or on CT of the head to expand the soft palate inferiorly and/or medially (Figure 2-12). Malignant neoplasms generally invade bone and interrupted bone cortices may be seen on bone windows. Benign masses may remodel bone but leave the cortices intact.

◆ KEY POINTS ◆

1. Squamous cell carcinoma is the most common type of head and neck cancer.

2. Contrast-enhanced CT and MRI each have advantages for assessment of head and neck cancer.

3. Disruption of normal anatomic spaces and vascular relationships is a useful finding when surveying the extent and origin of a tumor.

3

Neurologic Imaging

ANATOMY AND GENERAL PRINCIPLES

Like head and neck pathology, the differential diagnosis for intracranial and intraspinal lesions is determined by both anatomic location and imaging characteristics. A neoplasm in the posterior fossa has a different diagnostic approach than one in the middle cranial fossa or suprasellar region. Anatomically intracranial pathology is defined as either intra- or extra-axial, which is the first step in narrowing the differential diagnosis. The term intra-axial refers to any lesion within the brain parenchyma. Extra-axial refers to a lesion outside the brain parenchyma itself and may be between any layer of the meninges. Along the same line of reasoning, lesions within the spinal canal are classified as intramedullary, intradural, or extradural. Important imaging characteristics in neuroradiology include lesion size, shape, attenuation on CT, and signal characteristics on MRI. Contrast enhancement is an important characteristic for both modalities.

CT and MRI comprise the majority of neuroradiologic exams. Plain films are rarely used except for suspected skull fractures and occasional screening studies of the paranasal sinuses. CT is an effective screening exam for intracranial pathology, especially in trauma and emergent situations, because it has a high sensitivity for detecting acute bleeding and fractures and can be performed and interpreted rapidly. A CT exam is completed within a few minutes, whereas an MRI may require anywhere from 30 minutes to several hours to complete.

MRI is superior to CT in many situations, including evaluation of the posterior fossa, the detection of subtle lesions that are not associated with hemorrhage or significant edema, and spinal cord lesions. MR angiography (MRA) is also a useful, non-invasive technique to survey the intracranial vasculature for vascular malformations and aneurysms. MRI and MRA are often used for follow-up examinations when a head CT is abnormal. Images are acquired in multiple planes (axial, sagittal, and coronal) as opposed to CT, which is

---

◆ KEY POINTS ◆

1. The differential diagnosis for intracranial and intraspinal lesions is determined by both anatomic location and imaging characteristics.

2. Intra-axial refers to any lesion within the brain or spinal cord parenchyma and extra-axial refers to any lesion outside the brain parenchyma.

3. CT is ideal for emergency situations because it has a high sensitivity and can be performed and interpreted rapidly.

4. MRI generally has a higher specificity for intracranial abnormalities, as it detects subtle pathology in the brain and cerebral vasculature.

5. MRI produces images in multiple planes (axial, sagittal, and coronal).

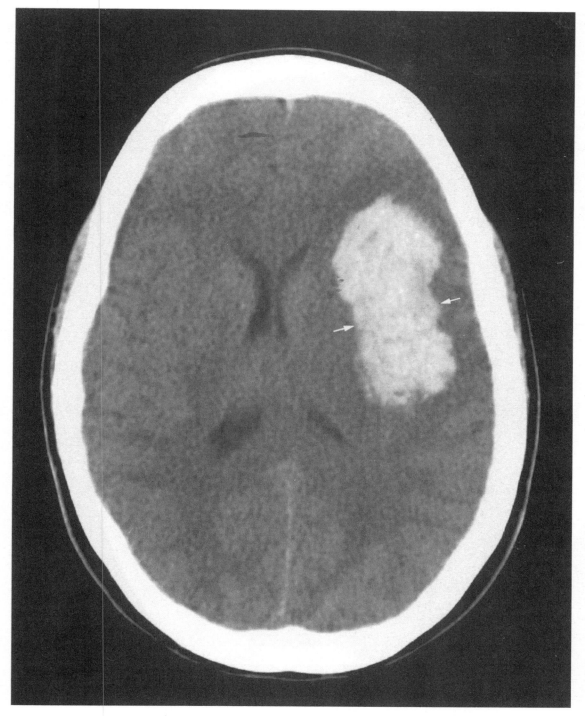

Figure 3-3. Intracerebral hematoma. This noncontrast CT image demonstrates blood within the left frontal lobe, which originated from an arteriovenous malformation. The patient presented with confusion and right hemiplegia. (Used with permission of Cedars-Sinai Medical Center, Los Angeles, California.)

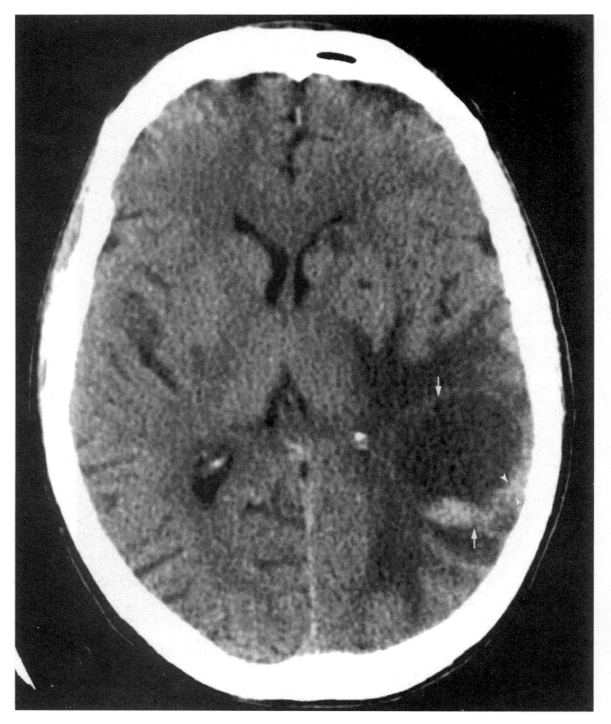

Figure 3-4. Metastatic lesion with hemorrhage. Non-contrast CT of the brain demonstrates a 4 cm left posterior parietal cystic mass (arrows) with areas of hemorrhage (arrowheads) and surrounding cytotoxic edema. This patient had a history of renal cell carcinoma and the lesion was a metastasis. (Used with permission of Cedars-Sinai Medical Center, Los Angeles, California.)

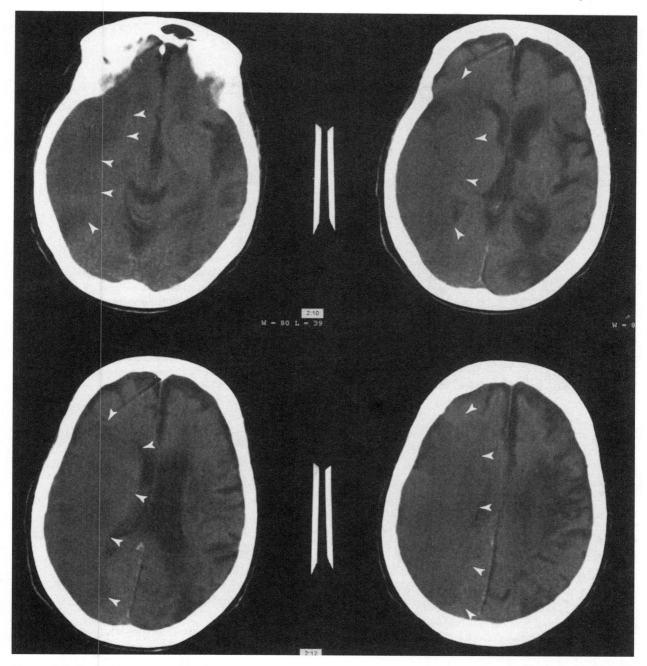

Figure 3-5. Stroke. Noncontrast CT of the brain demonstrates a large area of hypoattenuation spans the distribution of the right middle cerebral artery (MCA). A prior left MCA infarct with encephalomalacia is also present. (Used with permission of Cedars-Sinai Medical Center, Los Angeles, California.)

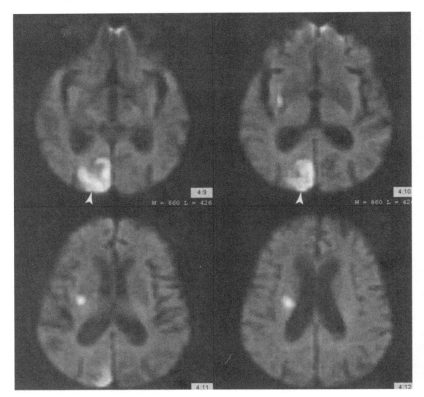

Figure 3-6. Stroke. MRI with diffusion-weighted imaging (DWI) reveals an area of high signal intensity in the right occipital lobe consistent with acute infarct in the right posterior cerebral artery distribution. (Used with permission of Cedars-Sinai Medical Center, Los Angeles, California.)

imaging study in suspected cases of stroke. It is important to exclude associated intracerebral hemorrhage, which would preclude anti-thrombotic treatment. Within a few hours, subtle findings emerge including loss of a distinct grey-white junction and blurring of the cortical sulci in the affected vascular distribution. Following thromboembolic strokes, low attenuation areas of edema within a vascular territory define the culprit vessel (Figure 3-5). Potential complications of stroke include delayed hemorrhage in the infarcted tissue, mass effect from the associated edema, and herniation with permanent brain damage or death. MRI with diffusion-weighted imaging (DWI) is a highly sensitive and specific test for cerebral infarction in the first six hours. DWI reveals bright signal intensity in the affected territory of the stroke (Figure 3-6).

◆ KEY POINTS ◆

1. Most cases of stroke are caused by thromboemboli.
2. Early in a stroke, the non-contrast CT of the brain will likely appear normal.
3. If a stroke is suspected, it is important to exclude an intracranial hemorrhage.
4. Loss of a distinct gray-white junction and blurring of the cortical sulci in the affected vascular distribution are subtle findings that appear within several hours.
5. MRI with diffusion-weighted imaging (DWI) is a highly sensitive and specific test for stroke.

4

Thoracic Imaging

ANATOMY AND GENERAL PRINCIPLES

The single most common diagnostic imaging exam today remains the chest radiograph. Every physician should develop a systematic approach to reading it. First, confirm the name of the patient, then determine the projection of the film. In the posterior-anterior (PA) projection (Figure 4-1a), the patient's chest is closer to the film compared to the anterior-posterior (AP) projection, where the patient's back is closer to the film. In the PA view, the clavicles appear slightly lower on the film, the scapulae project more laterally, and the posterior elements of the vertebral bodies are more clearly visualized than on an AP film. The PA projection is preferred because the heart is closer to the film and is less magnified and its size more accurately displayed. The lateral film (Figure 4-1b) is generally used in conjunction with the PA film, and provides more information about cardiac enlargement, pleural effusions, location of lung parenchymal pathology, and position of mediastinal masses.

For an adequate PA radiograph, the patient must be able to stand or sit in a wheelchair. If the patient is too unstable or too ill to come to the imaging department for the PA film, an AP radiograph is obtained using a portable x-ray machine (Figure 4-1c). The next step in reading a chest radiograph is using a systematic approach to evaluate the five essential areas of the film:

1) **Air:** lungs, including central airways and pulmonary vessels

2) **Bones:** ribs, clavicles, spine, shoulders, and scapulae

3) **Cardiac:** heart and mediastinum

4) **Diaphragm** and pleural surfaces

5) **Everything** else: lines and tubes, upper abdomen, soft tissues of chest wall and neck

With a systematic approach used on every exam, nothing on the film is left uninspected. First, the lungs should normally be the darkest portions of the film, as the air within the alveoli is easily penetrated by the x-ray beam. The lungs will span approximately nine to 10 posterior ribs or seven to eight anterior ribs in a normal inspiration. The pulmonary vessels are normally seen radiating from the hila, with gradual tapering to the periphery. The normal distribution of the pulmonary vessels is two-thirds of the blood flow to the lower portions of the lungs and one-third to the upper lobes. The lungs are scrutinized for focal areas of abnormality, such as atelectasis, masses, or nodules and then for diffuse processes such as alveolar or interstitial patterns. An alveolar or "airspace" pattern is a confluent opacification, often confined to one lobe or lobar segment, as in pneumonia. Air normally found in the alveoli has been replaced by more radio-opaque material such as pus, water, blood, cells, or proteinaceous material. An interstitial pattern is often described as a lace-like or "reticular."

The next area of focus is the skeleton, with inspection of the osseous structures described previously. Particular

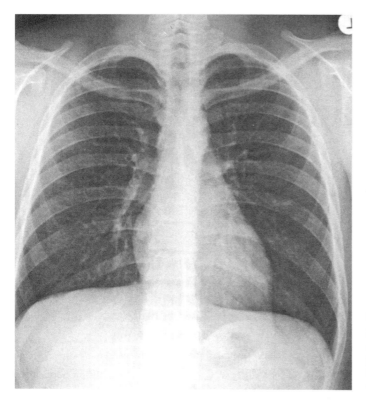

Figure 4-1a. Normal posterior-anterior (PA) chest radiograph. (Used with permission of Cedars-Sinai Medical Center, Los Angeles, California.)

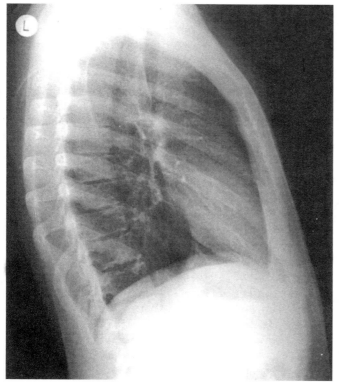

Figure 4-1b. Normal lateral chest radiograph. (Used with permission of Cedars-Sinai Medical Center, Los Angeles, California.)

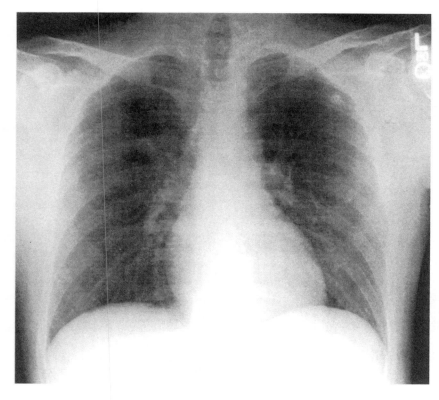

Figure 4-1c. Normal portable anterior-posterior (AP) chest radiograph. (Used with permission of Cedars-Sinai Medical Center, Los Angeles, California.)

attention is given to the ribs and spine for fractures and metastatic lesions, and the shoulders for evidence of arthritis.

Evaluation of the cardiac silhouette and mediastinum is crucial for interpretation of the chest radiograph. The mediastinum is divided into anterior, middle, and posterior sections as seen on a lateral chest radiograph. The anterior mediastinum includes the anterior chest wall to the anterior heart border. Pathology that may be found here includes the "four Ts": thyroid masses, thymoma, teratoma, and "terrible lymphoma." The middle mediastinum includes the heart, hilar structures, esophagus, and descending aorta. Common pathologies in this area include lymph node enlargement, hiatal hernia, descending aortic aneurysm, and esophageal pathology. The posterior mediastinum on the lateral radiograph includes the thoracic vertebral bodies and paravertebral soft tissues.

In the frontal (PA or AP) projections of the chest, several landmarks of the mediastinum are useful in finding pathology. On the right side of the mediastinum, there are three convexities or "moguls."

From superior to inferior, these are the superior vena cava, ascending aorta, and right atrium. On the left margin of the mediastinum, the three convexities are the aortic arch, pulmonary artery outflow tract, and left ventricle. Between the left-sided moguls, there are normally two concavities: the aortopulmonary window and the region of the left atrial appendage. If either of these two concavities is replaced by soft tissue, the mediastinum is abnormal and further work-up is required.

When lung pathology is found, an effort should be made to describe its location, including the lobe and, if possible, the segment. One method of making this determination is to look for areas that are silhouetted or obscured by the pathology. For example, any lesion that obscures the right or left heart border must be in either the right middle lobe or the lingula respectively. If either hemidiaphragm is silhouetted, the pathology is in the adjacent lower lobe.

Another general principle in reading chest radiographs is making a determination of the predominant pattern in the lungs. Certain patterns may suggest specific diseases, but, more often, the patterns overlap, i.e., granulomatous disease of the lung may mimic metastatic lung nodules. One should also keep in mind the broad categories into which pathologic processes can be classified. One mnemonic is "MACHINE": metabolic, autoimmune, congenital, hematologic, infectious, neoplastic, and environmental. Of course, some pathology will not fit into these groups, but a majority will, and reviewing the list each time will be helpful in generating a differential diagnosis.

One way to avoid common errors is to avoid the temptation to evaluate a chest film with a "quick glance." Sometimes when the main finding on the film is discovered, the remainder of the systematic approach is abandoned, and secondary findings may be missed. This type of mistake is commonly referred to as a "satisfaction of search" error.

◆ KEY POINTS ◆

1. The chest radiograph is the most common imaging study.

2. A systematic approach with evaluation of the air, bones, cardiac shadow, diaphragm, and everything else is essential in the interpretation of any chest film.

3. Alveolar opacification of the lungs represents blood, water, or pus in the acute phase and either cells or protein in the chronic stage.

4. When pathology is found, complete a thorough evaluation of the film to avoid the "satisfaction of search" error.

INFECTION

Lobar Pneumonia

History

Patients with lobar pneumonia present with chief complaints of fever, productive cough, and shortness of breath. Symptoms generally start gradually and worsen over two to four days. Some patients complain of chest pain or abdominal pain in some cases of lower lobe pneumonia.

Physical Examination

Dullness to percussion, egophony, and tactile fremitus are classic physical findings with lobar consolidation. Rales are often heard over the affected segments. If the lung is consolidated and air cannot penetrate into the alveoli, decreased breath sounds are noted.

Radiographic Findings

The radiologic appearance of pneumonia varies depending on several factors including: the type of pathogen (whether bacterial, viral, fungal, or atypical), underlying lung disease (COPD, chronic interstitial lung disease, cystic fibrosis), and risk factors for the patient (aspiration risk, immunocompromise, TB exposure).

Most cases of bacterial pneumonia have the common appearance of alveolar opacification in a lobar distribution on chest radiograph (Figure 4-2a, b). Common pathogens are *Streptococcus pneumoniae*, *Haemophilus influenzae*, *Klebsiella pneumoniae*, and *Neisseria meningitidis*. The process may affect an entire lobe and demonstrate a sharp border with the adjacent lobe, or only involve specific segments of a lobe. Some radiologists compare the appearance of alveolar opacification to a patchy fog overlying the film. Often air-bronchograms are seen, which are evident because air remains in the bronchi and is surrounded by densely consolidated adjacent lung tissue, creating an air-tissue interface. The air-tissue interface is evident on the radiograph because of the differences in attenuation (Figure 4-2a, b). It must be noted however, that air bronchograms are nonspecific and do not equate exclusively with pneumonia. They only demonstrate that the process is within the lung parenchyma, not in the pleural space or overlying soft tissue. Usually there is little or no associated volume loss with lobar pneumonia because the bronchi are air-filled and do not collapse.

◆ KEY POINTS ◆

1. Bacterial pneumonia is commonly caused by *Streptococcus pneumoniae*, *Haemophilus influenzae*, *Klebsiella pneumoniae*, and *Neisseria meningitidis*.

2. Alveolar opacification in a lobar distribution on chest radiograph is the classic radiographic finding for bacterial pneumonia.

3. Alveolar opacification looks like a patchy fog overlying the film.

4. Air-bronchograms are common in lobar pneumonia.

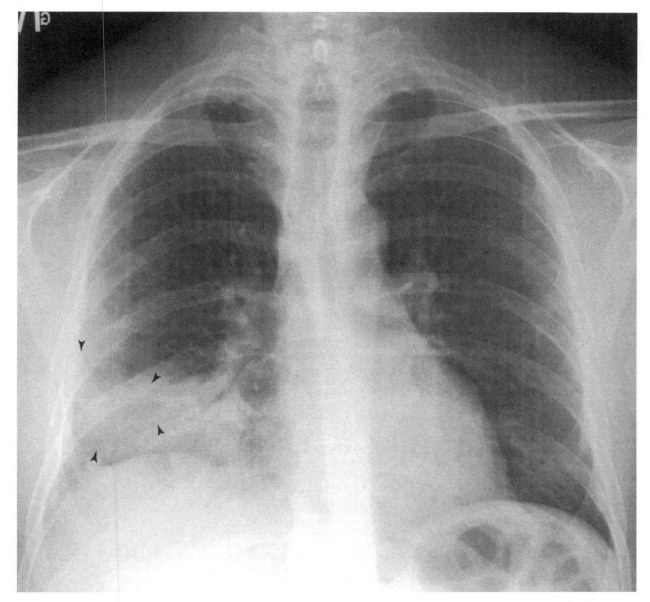

Figure 4-2a. Lobar pneumonia on PA chest radiograph. There is alveolar opacification in the lateral segment of the right middle lobe. (Used with permission of Cedars-Sinai Medical Center, Los Angeles, California.)

Bronchopneumonia

Pathophysiology

As opposed to lobar pneumonia, which affects the alveoli, bronchopneumonia primarily affects the bronchi, bronchioles, and some scattered adjacent alveoli. There may be evidence of volume loss as the bronchi become inflamed and filled with pus and the distal alveoli collapse. Common pathogens include Staphylococcus aureus, Gram negatives and in some cases of *Mycoplasma pneumoniae* (which may also present with an interstitial pattern).

Radiographic Findings

Patchy opacification in a segmental as opposed to a lobar distribution is common with bronchopneumonia (Figure 4-3). Air bronchograms are not present as in

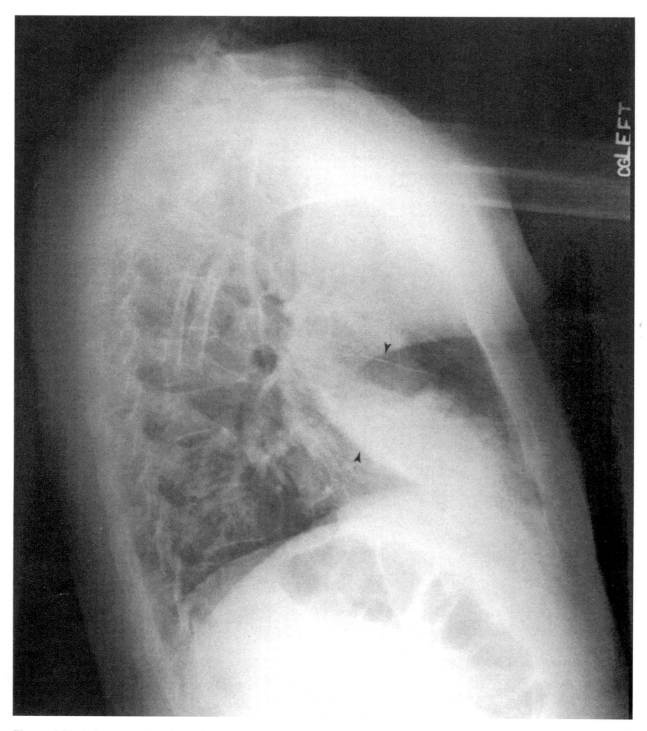

Figure 4-2b. Lobar pneumonia. Lateral view in the same patient as Figure 4-2a with alveolar opacification outlining the borders of the right middle lobe. (Used with permission of Cedars-Sinai Medical Center, Los Angeles, California.)

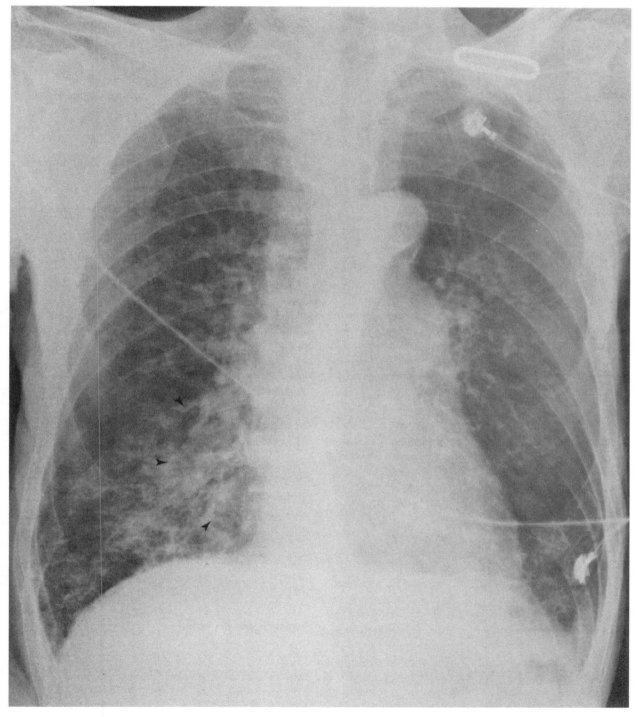

Figure 4-3. Bronchopneumonia. There is patchy alveolar opacification of the right middle lobe with silhouetting of the right heart border. This 88-year old patient had silent aspiration on a video swallowing study and the findings represent aspiration pneumonia. (Used with permission of Cedars-Sinai Medical Center, Los Angeles, California.)

lobar pneumonia because the bronchi are filled with exudate and there is no air-tissue interface to delineate them.

◆ **KEY POINTS** ◆

1. Bronchopneumonia causes patchy opacification on chest radiograph due to collapse of distal alveoli.
2. Air bronchograms are usually not present as with lobar pneumonia.

Asthma
Pathophysiology

The pathophysiology of asthma involves hyperreactive airway mucosa, low threshold for the degranulation of mast cells in response to irritants, and increased IgE. As the airway mucosa becomes edematous, and there is spasm of the bronchial smooth muscle, the lumen narrows and the result is decreased air movement. The effect is mostly on the bronchioles and smaller airways, but all central airways may be involved.

History and Physical

Patients complain of shortness of breath and wheezing, and sometimes cough. Prolonged expiration, decreased breath sounds, expiratory wheezes, and accessory muscle use for resting respiration are common physical findings.

Radiographic Findings

Radiographically, most patients with asthma will have a normal chest x-ray. However, there may be evidence of hyperinflated lungs (Figure 4-4a), atelectasis, and peribronchial cuffing (Figure 4-4b). Hyperinflated lungs are determined by an inspiratory result that demonstrates more than 10 posterior ribs above the diaphragm, often with an increased retrosternal air space seen on the lateral view. Peribronchial cuffing is the radiographic manifestation of edema surrounding the bronchial tree. It is a nonspecific finding which may be seen in other lung processes such as chronic bronchitis, bronchiectasis, pulmonary edema, and cystic fibrosis. Taking into consideration the patient's past medical history can help in distinguishing these.

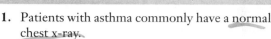

◆ **KEY POINTS** ◆

1. Patients with asthma commonly have a normal chest x-ray.
2. Hyperinflated lungs, peribronchial inflammation, and atelectasis are nonspecific, associated radiographic findings with asthma.

Neoplasm
Epidemiology

It is essential to define the location of a lung neoplasm as parenchymal, mediastinal, or pleural-based because the clinical presentations, differential diagnoses, and treatments differ for each. Smoking is the greatest risk factor for lung neoplasm and approximately 92% of patients with lung cancer have a history of smoking. From another point of view, 10% of all heavy smokers (more than 35 pack-years) will develop lung cancer. The most common type of cancer found in smokers is squamous cell carcinoma followed by adenocarcinoma. Often lung cancer will metastasize. Common sites of metastasis are liver, adrenal glands, distant lung parenchyma, brain, and, less commonly, bone. Cancers which commonly metastasize *to* the lungs are breast, renal, colon, testicular, melanomas, and sarcomas.

Bronchogenic Carcinoma
Epidemiology

The term bronchogenic carcinoma is a broad classification that defines a neoplasm that arises within a bronchus but includes several different cell types. Examples of bronchogenic lesions include adenocarcinoma (45%), squamous cell carcinoma (35%), small cell carcinoma (15%), and large cell carcinoma (1–5%).

Radiographic Findings

The appearance of adenocarcinoma on plain film and CT is that of a peripheral mass (>5 cm) or nodule (<5 cm) often with spiculated borders (Figures 4-5a, b, c). There is a subtype of adenocarcinoma, namely bronchioloalveolar carcinoma, which has a different radiographic appearance. Bronchioloalveolar carcinoma may present as multiple nodules, with chronic airspace consolidation, or as an interstitial pattern as the tumor

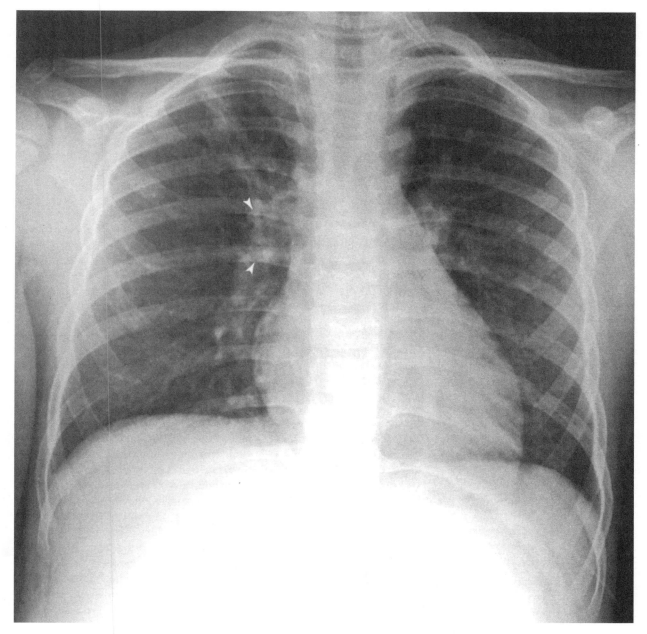

Figure 4-4a. Asthma. AP chest radiograph demonstrates hyperinflated lungs and peribronchial cuffing or edema surrounding the medium-sized airways. (Used with permission of Cedars-Sinai Medical Center, Los Angeles, California.)

cells grow along the interstitial framework of the lung producing a "lepidic" or "scale-like" pattern.

Squamous cell carcinoma tends to occur within the walls of a central bronchus and present with bronchial obstruction and associated atelectasis of the corresponding lobe. Small cell carcinoma also usually presents as a central mass. Large cell carcinoma can be located centrally or peripherally.

A contrast-enhanced CT scan of the chest is the next appropriate test in the assessment of a known

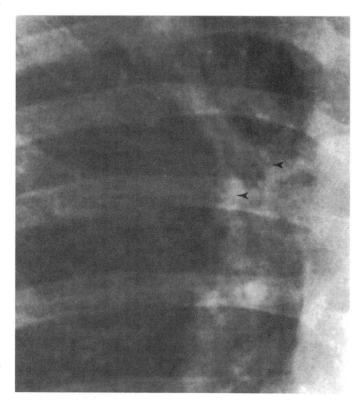

Figure 4-4b. Asthma. Magnification of right upper lobe bronchi with peribronchial edema. (Used with permission of Cedars-Sinai Medical Center, Los Angeles, California.)

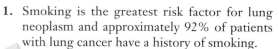

◆ KEY POINTS ◆

1. Smoking is the greatest risk factor for lung neoplasm and approximately 92% of patients with lung cancer have a history of smoking.

2. The most common type of cancer found in smokers is squamous cell carcinoma, followed by adenocarcinoma.

3. The classic appearance of adenocarcinoma on plain film and CT is that of a peripheral mass or nodule with spiculated borders.

4. Squamous cell carcinoma tends to occur within the walls of a central bronchus and present with bronchial obstruction and associated atelectasis of the corresponding lobe.

5. A contrast-enhanced CT scan of the chest is the next appropriate test in the assessment of a known pulmonary mass.

pulmonary mass. Today's CT scanners detect nodules as small as 0.3 cm with consistency. Associated findings include ipsilateral mediastinal lymphadenopathy, malignant pleural effusions containing neoplastic cells, and atelectasis or post-obstructive pneumonia from a lesion that occludes a bronchus. Lymph nodes are best seen using soft tissue window and level settings and are considered pathologic if they are larger than 1 cm in the shortest axis. A different appearance is seen with bronchoalveolar carcinoma, which may have a chronic airspace consolidation pattern similar to common pneumonia. Cavitation of a lesion is most commonly seen with squamous cell carcinoma and may help in distinguishing it from the other causes of neoplastic masses.

Metastases

Pathophysiology

Primary cancers from extrapulmonary sources may metastasize to the lungs by two main mechanisms:

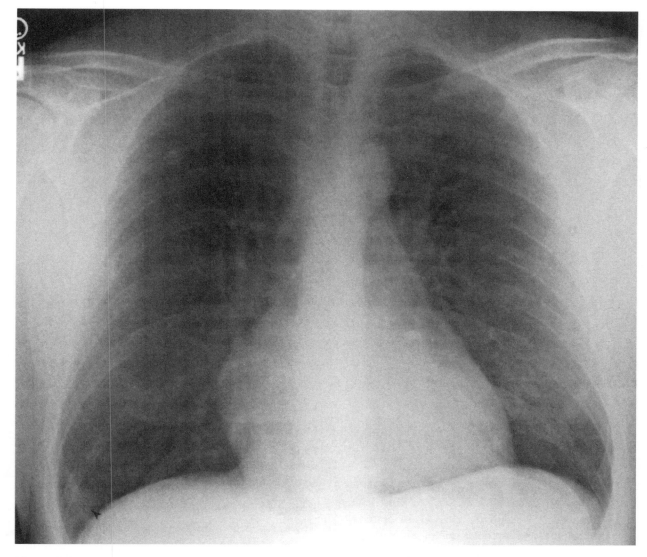

Figure 4-5a. Adenocarcinoma of the lung. PA chest radiograph with right lower lobe peripheral nodule near the right costophrenic angle. (Used with permission of Cedars-Sinai Medical Center, Los Angeles, California.)

hematogenous spread through the systemic circulation via the pulmonary arterial blood supply and lymphatic spread via the periaortic and celiac lymph nodes to the posterior mediastinal lymph nodes.

Common sources of hematogenous spread are vascular neoplasms such as renal cell carcinoma, thyroid carcinoma, melanoma, and sarcomas. Common neoplasms that exhibit lymphatic spread are breast, gastric, pancreatic, laryngeal, and cervical carcinomas.

Radiographic Appearance

Almost exclusively, hematogenous lung metastases appear as multiple, variably sized lesions with sharp, round margins (Figure 4-6a, b). They have a propensity for the lung bases more than the apices, due to the relative increase in blood flow in the bases. Metastases from lymphatic spread have a higher percentage of solitary mass lesions at presentation but may also have multiple discrete nodules. Associated mediastinal lymphadenopathy

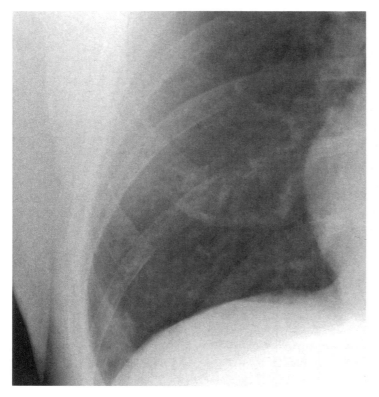

Figure 4-5b. Adenocarcinoma of the lung. Magnification of lung nodule in Figure 4-5a shows subtle poorly demarcated nodule. (Used with permission of Cedars-Sinai Medical Center, Los Angeles, California.)

is common with both hematogenous and lymphatic metastatic neoplasms.

◆ KEY POINTS ◆

1. Renal cell carcinoma, thyroid carcinoma, melanoma, and sarcomas commonly metastasize to the lungs by hematogenous spread.
2. The classic radiographic appearance of lung metastases is multiple, well demarcated pulmonary nodules.

Sarcoidosis

Epidemiology

Sarcoidosis is a chronic, multisystem granulomatous disease of uncertain etiology. The disease is 10 to 20 times more common in blacks than whites and usually occurs in the third to fifth decades of life.

History

Patients with pulmonary involvement usually present with a cough or with dyspnea. The lung is involved somewhat in approximately 90% of cases.

Radiographic Findings

Radiographically, pulmonary sarcoidosis appears in stages. Stage 0 occurs before there is radiographic evidence of the disease as an essentially normal film. The diagnosis of sarcoidosis may have been made based on involvement of other organs such as the skin, eyes, liver, or spleen. Hepatosplenomegaly is found in 15 to 20% of all cases. Only 10% of patients will present with stage 0. Stage 1 pulmonary sarcoidosis demonstrates bilateral symmetric hilar lymphadenopathy, and represents 50% of cases (Figure 4-7a, b). Patients present with a nonproductive cough, as the adenopathy initiates a cough reflex. Stage 2 sarcoidosis has bilateral hilar lymphadenopathy, but also demonstrates reticulonodular parenchymal opacities. Some nodules may reach 1 cm in size and the initial

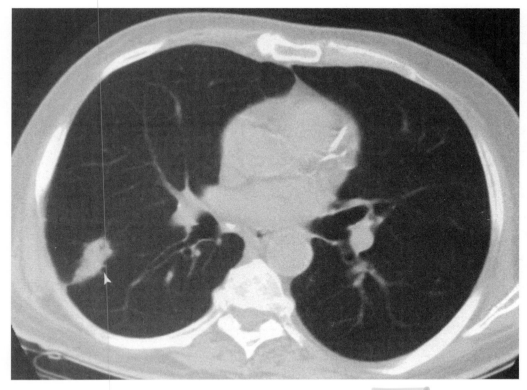

Figure 4-5c. Adenocarcinoma on CT of the chest with lung windows. A spiculated, peripheral soft tissue mass is seen in the right lower lobe. (Used with permission of Cedars-Sinai Medical Center, Los Angeles, California.)

pattern may progress to appear as patchy consolidation with air bronchograms. As the disease progresses, stage 3 sarcoidosis presents increased pulmonary parenchymal opacities but the lymphadenopathy decreases. It is as though the disease process moves out of the hilar lymph nodes into the lungs. Stage 4 represents end-stage disease with pulmonary fibrosis and bullae formation with upper lobe predominance.

Chest radiographs are useful for initial diagnosis and monitoring treatment. Chest CT is best for defining the extent of lymphadenopathy at stage 1 and for early detection of progression to stage 2 with interstitial disease. High-resolution CT is useful during stage 2 sarcoidosis, as interstitial disease is more evident compared to standard chest CT imaging. A nuclear medicine gallium scan will demonstrate increased uptake in the hilar lymph nodes during active stage 1 disease. It is less sensitive once the process has moved from the hila to the lung parenchyma.

◆ KEY POINTS ◆

1. Sarcoidosis is a chronic granulomatous disease.

2. Bilateral hilar lymph node enlargement is the classic, though nonspecific, early radiographic finding.

3. Sarcoidosis may progress to involve the lung parenchyma to cause interstitial fibrosis in stage 4 disease.

Cardiomegaly

Anatomy

When looking at a PA chest radiograph it is common to measure the apparent diameter of the heart and

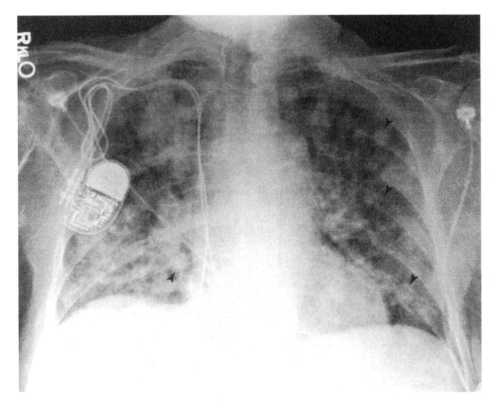

Figure 4-6a. Lung metastases. AP chest radiograph with numerous, round, well-demarcated metastatic nodules. (Used with permission of Cedars-Sinai Medical Center, Los Angeles, California.)

compare it to the span of the chest at the level of the dome of the right hemidiaphragm. If this ratio is greater than one-half, then the cardiac silhouette is enlarged (Figure 4-8). The term "cardiac silhouette" includes the contribution of the pericardium and not just the heart itself. If a large pericardial effusion is present, the cardiac silhouette will appear enlarged even if the heart itself is normal in size. It would be incorrect to use the term "cardiomegaly" in this case. Measurement of the cardiac silhouette is not accurate on the portable AP radiograph because there is a magnification effect due to the heart's increased distance from the film. The cardiac silhouette will always appear slightly larger on an AP film than it truly measures.

Pathophysiology

Causes of an enlarged cardiac silhouette and more specifically cardiomegaly include ischemic cardiomyopathy, hypertension, valvular disease, congenital heart disease, and several other less common conditions such as viral cardiomyopathy and cardiac mass lesions.

By far the most common cause of cardiomegaly is ischemic cardiomyopathy or congestive heart failure. It is the inability of the heart muscle to keep pace with forward blood flow, in other words, pump failure. This may occur when the cardiac muscle is "stunned" by an acute ischemic event following a myocardial infarct or it may occur later when there is decreased wall motion in the territory of a coronary artery with a stenosis or occlusion.

Radiographic Findings

The PA film is more useful than an AP radiograph for determining cardiomegaly because the heart is closer to the film and its size is more accurate. A lateral radiograph will yield information as to specific chamber enlargement (Figure 4-9). The left atrium sits

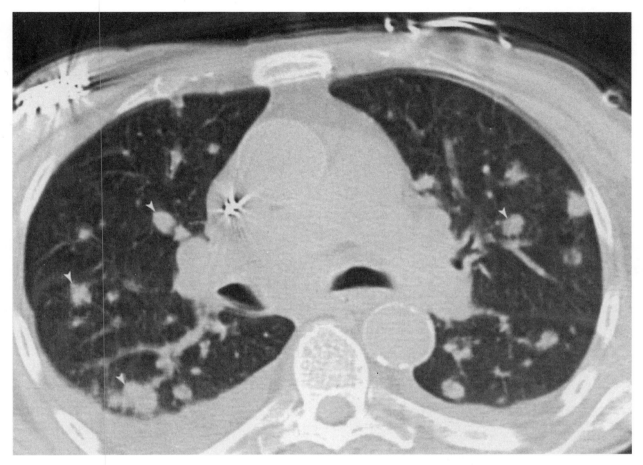

Figure 4-6b. Lung metastases. CT of the same patient in Figure 4-6a demonstrating numerous metastatic nodules. (Used with permission of Cedars-Sinai Medical Center, Los Angeles, California.)

posteriorly on the lateral view and may be seen to bulge towards the spine if enlarged. Left ventricular enlargement appears as a rounded left cardiac border and with downward displacement of the cardiac apex on the PA view.

◆ KEY POINTS ◆

1. The PA chest film is more useful than an AP radiograph for determining cardiomegaly because the heart is closer to the film and therefore the heart size is more accurate.

2. The lateral film is often useful for determining specific chamber enlargement.

Pulmonary Edema

Etiology

Pulmonary edema occurs in a variety of processes. Most commonly, it is seen with left-sided heart failure, aortic stenosis, and renal failure with total body fluid overload. Another less common category is lung injury that includes adult respiratory distress syndrome (ARDS), sepsis, aspiration, and inhalation injuries.

Radiographic Findings

Radiographic features of cardiogenic pulmonary edema can be graded according to severity. Grade I demonstrates upper lung pulmonary vascular congestion where the normal distribution of pulmonary venous

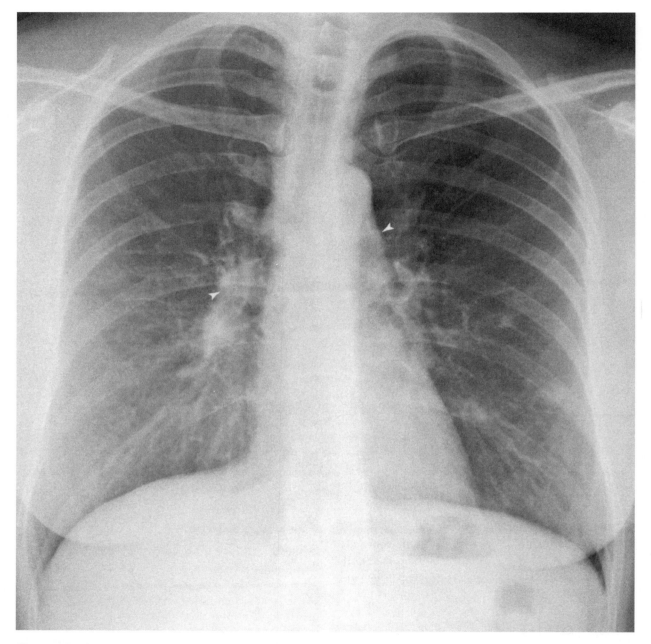

Figure 4-7a. Sarcoidosis. Bilateral hilar lymph node enlargement on PA chest radiograph. (Used with permission of Cedars-Sinai Medical Center, Los Angeles, California.)

blood flow of one third to upper lobes and two thirds to lower lobes is altered. In most cases, the distribution becomes more half to half as evidenced by increased diameter of the upper lobe pulmonary veins. In grade 2 cardiogenic pulmonary edema, the radiograph shows peribronchial cuffing, pleural effusions and Kerley B lines, which represent interstitial edema. Grade 3 edema has the addition of alveolar opacification,

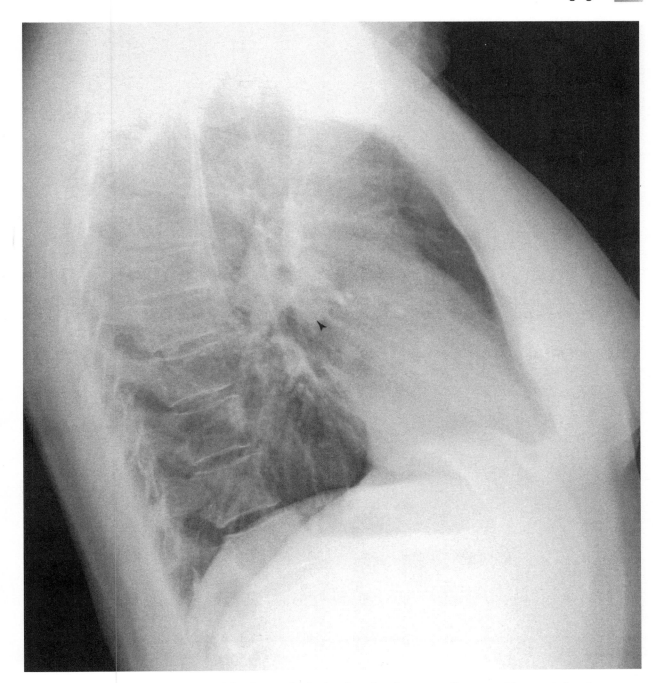

Figure 4-7b. Sarcoidosis. Lateral view of the chest with hilar lymph node enlargement. Compare with normal chest in Figure 4-1b. (Used with permission of Cedars-Sinai Medical Center, Los Angeles, California.)

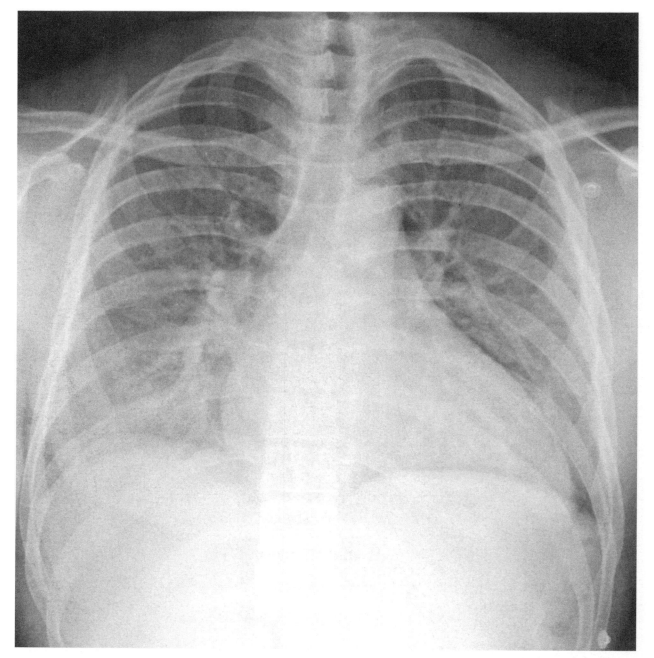

Figure 4-8. Cardiomegaly. PA chest radiograph demonstrating enlargement of the cardiac silhouette which spans more than one-half the diameter of the chest. (Used with permission of Cedars-Sinai Medical Center, Los Angeles, California.)

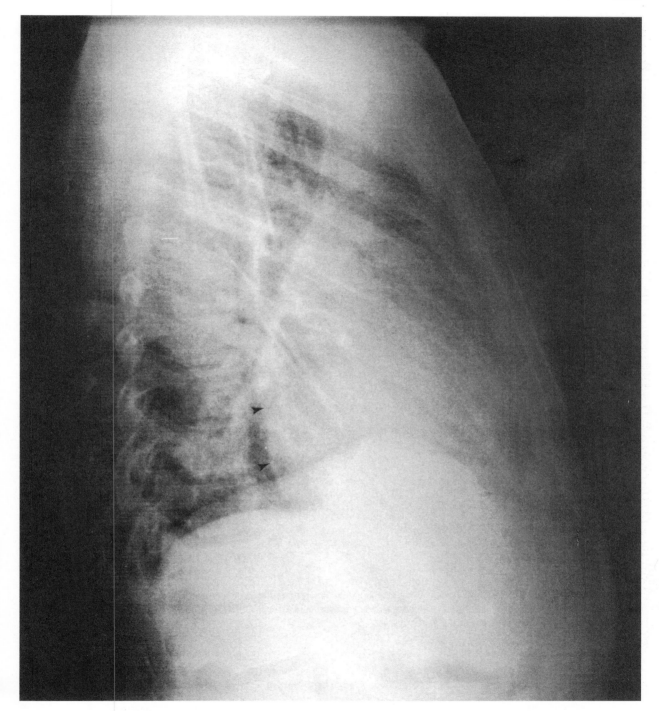

Figure 4-9. Cardiomegaly. Lateral view. Lateral radiograph of the patient in Figure 4-8 demonstrates cardiomegaly with enlargement of the left atrium, with the posterior border of the heart nearly reaching the spine. (Used with permission of Cedars-Sinai Medical Center, Los Angeles, California.)

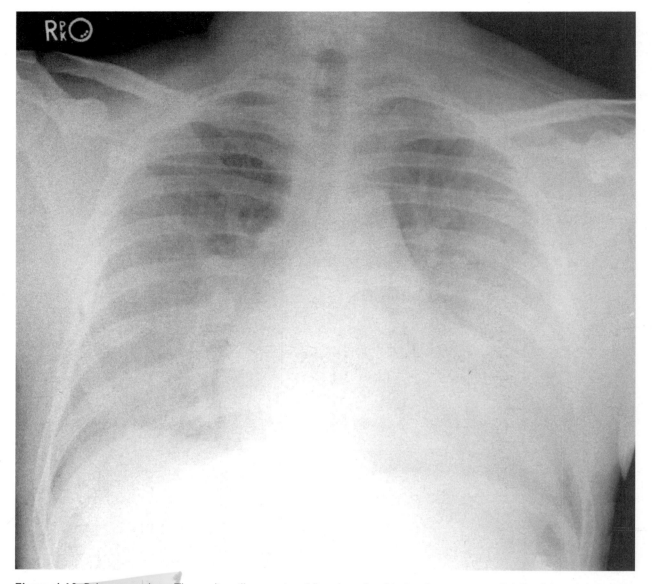

Figure 4-10. Pulmonary edema. The cardiac silhouette is mildly enlarged and its borders are not well defined due to the overlying alveolar opacification from edema. The patient had a massive myocardial infarction and flash pulmonary edema. (Used with permission of Cedars-Sinai Medical Center, Los Angeles, California.)

especially in the lung bases and perihilar region (Figure 4-10). Air bronchograms may be seen as the alveoli are filled with water and the bronchi contain air, causing an air-water interface. Decompensated aortic stenosis has similar findings, in the setting of cardiac enlargement and elevated left atrial pressures measured with a Swan-Ganz catheter.

Non-cardiogenic pulmonary edema is most often associated with renal failure and volume overload. It is common with patients on dialysis. The radiographic appearance is different from cardiogenic pulmonary edema in several ways. First, the heart size is usually normal unless there is also a cardiac comorbidity. Next, the alveolar opacification usually occurs

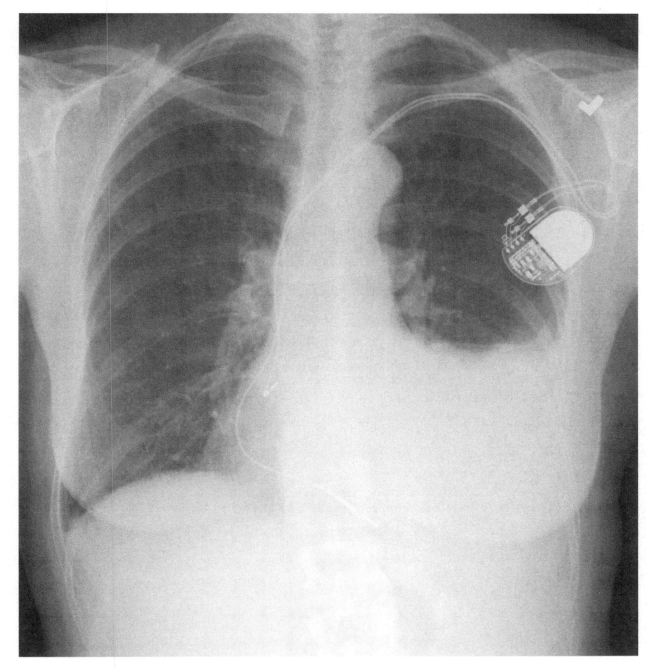

Figure 4-11. Pleural effusion. PA chest radiograph showing a moderate-sized left pleural effusion which effaces the left costophrenic angle and left diaphragm. (Used with permission of Cedars-Sinai Medical Center, Los Angeles, California.)

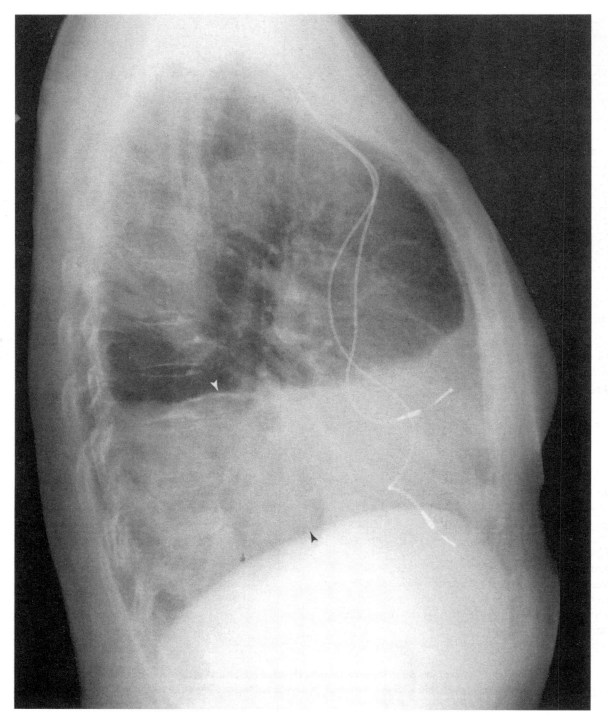

Figure 4-12. Pleural effusion. Lateral view. White arrowhead shows top of pleural effusion. Black arrowhead is the contralateral (right) hemidiaphragm. The left hemidiaphragm is silhouetted by the pleural fluid. (Used with permission of Cedars-Sinai Medical Center, Los Angeles, California.)

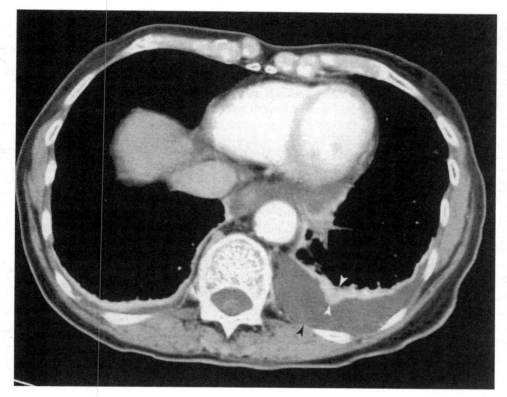

Figure 4-13. Pleural effusion. CT scan of the chest with soft tissue windowing. There is a small left pleural effusion (black arrowhead) and adjacent atelectasis (white arrowheads). (Used with permission of Cedars-Sinai Medical Center, Los Angeles, California.)

centrally in a perihilar distribution and air bronchograms are infrequently seen. The pulmonary venous blood flow is usually balanced 50% to each of the upper and lower lung zones. As with cardiogenic edema, pleural effusions and Kerley B lines are common.

Edema caused by pulmonary injury predominantly involves the alveoli. It is difficult to distinguish from non-cardiogenic pulmonary edema. As a reaction to the initial insult, the alveoli fill with fluid and exudate, causing patchy opacifications and air bronchograms. The heart size and pulmonary vessels are normal and Kerley B lines and pleural effusions are rarely seen.

Pleural Effusion

Pathophysiology

A pleural effusion represents an increase above the normal physiologic amount of fluid in the pleural space between the parietal and visceral pleura. It is nonspecific

---

◆ KEY POINTS ◆

1. Pulmonary edema is most commonly seen with left-sided heart failure, aortic stenosis, and renal failure with total body fluid overload.

2. Upper lung pulmonary vascular congestion is the earliest radiographic sign of pulmonary edema.

3. Kerley B lines, peribronchial fluid, and pleural effusions are classic signs of pulmonary vascular congestion and edema.

4. Alveolar opacification represents advanced pulmonary vascular congestion and defines true pulmonary edema.

---

and can be associated with many different pathologic processes. The most common causes are cardiogenic and noncardiogenic pulmonary edema, pneumonia, neoplasm, and autoimmune diseases. There are two categories of effusions; transudative and exudative. Transudative effusions are generally associated with congestive heart failure, cirrhosis, or protein-losing nephropathy. Exudative effusions are commonly associated with neoplastic processes and pneumonia.

Radiographic Findings

The radiographic features of a pleural effusion are "blunting" of the costophrenic angles on PA (Figure 4-11) and lateral (Figure 4-12) radiographs, fluid in the horizontal or minor fissures, or thickened pleura laterally or apically on an AP radiograph in a patient positioned more supine than upright or sitting. Lateral decubitus plain films are useful to determine whether the effusion is mobile and therefore can be aspirated during a thoracentesis. A CT scan of the chest will reveal the size of a pleural effusion (Figure 4-13), may identify loculations as separate, water-attenuation collections that do not layer along the dependent portion of the chest, and can distinguish pleural fluid from an adjacent parenchymal process such as atelectasis or pneumonia. Occasionally, the costophrenic angle may appear normal, but an effusion may still be present. This is referred to as a subpulmonic effusion and is characterized by fluid that lies between the inferior portion of the lung and the hemidiaphragm. A hint that there is a subpulmonic effusion is that the apex of the hemidiaphragm will appear to be located more lateral than normal on a PA film.

◆ KEY POINTS ◆

1. A pleural effusion is an increase above the normal physiologic amount of fluid in the pleural space between the parietal and visceral pleura.

2. The classic radiographic finding of a pleural effusion is "blunting" of the costophrenic angle, best seen on the lateral view.

3. Lateral decubitus plain films are useful to determine whether the effusion is mobile or loculated.

5

Abdominal Imaging

SMALL BOWEL OBSTRUCTION

Anatomy

The small bowel is divided into three main segments: the duodenum, jejunum, and ileum. On a kidneys, ureters, and bladder radiograph (KUB), the small bowel is sometimes seen as scattered gas bubbles throughout the abdomen. Each segment of the small bowel has a general location that helps to distinguish it from large bowel. The duodenum is the portion of intestine that forms a C-loop in the mid- and right upper abdomen, and is divided into four segments, from the duodenal bulb to the ligament of Treitz. The jejunum is a long segment of intestine coiled in the left upper abdomen that has thin, circular folds called "valvulae conniventes." These folds help to distinguish small bowel from large bowel, which have thicker, incomplete folds, called haustra. The ileum, located mostly in the mid- and right lower abdomen also has valvulae conniventes. It is the terminal portion of the small intestine, and is responsible for the absorption of bile salts and fat-soluble vitamins: A, D, E, K, and B12.

Etiology

A small bowel obstruction is defined as an interruption of the normal antegrade transit of intestinal contents. Obstructions are mechanical in nature; i.e., the force of antegrade flow is lower than that needed to move intestinal material through the point of obstruction. Obstructions may be partial, allowing some passage of intestinal contents, or complete. One of the most common causes is the formation of adhesions that form scar-like bands and constrict a portion of bowel. Adhesions sometimes occur after intra-abdominal surgery or in areas of prior inflammation. The second most common cause of small bowel obstruction is hernia. The two main classifications of hernia are abdominal wall and internal. Other causes of small bowel obstruction include neoplasm, intussusception, ischemia, volvulus, Crohn's disease, Meckel's diverticulum, gallstone ileus, and intramural hematoma.

Epidemiology

Patients who have had prior intra-abdominal surgery are at increased risk for obstruction due to the formation of adhesions. A hernia or intraluminal bowel mass may also be a lead point for obstruction. Any intra-abdominal neoplasm may encase bowel, leading to obstruction. Crohn's disease with stricture formation is a risk factor.

History

Patients present with abdominal pain, nausea, vomiting, and obstipation. Pain is often diffuse and crampy, occurring as peristalsis pushes against the obstruction at intervals of five to 15 minutes. Nausea and vomiting are most common in proximal small bowel obstruction, as the stomach and duodenum dilate early. Obstipation occurs as intestinal material does not pass into the colon. The fecal material present at the time of the obstruction may pass, but lack of flatus and bowel movements is an important portion of the history.

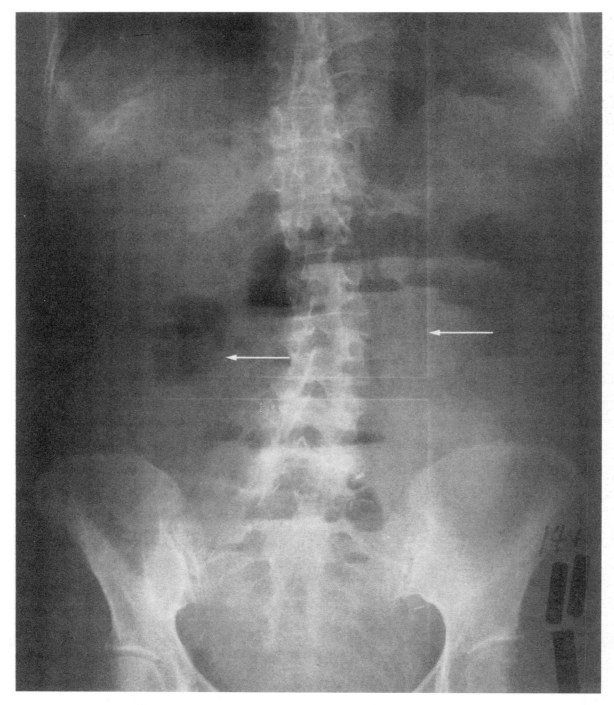

Figures 5-1, 5-2. Small bowel obstruction. Upright (5-1) and supine (5-2) KUB films demonstrate dilated air-filled loops of small bowel on the supine film and air-fluid levels on the upright film. This 60-year old female has a history of abdominal surgery for ovarian cancer debulking. The obstruction was due to adhesions that formed a few months after the surgery. (Used with permission of Cedars-Sinai Medical Center, Los Angeles, California.)

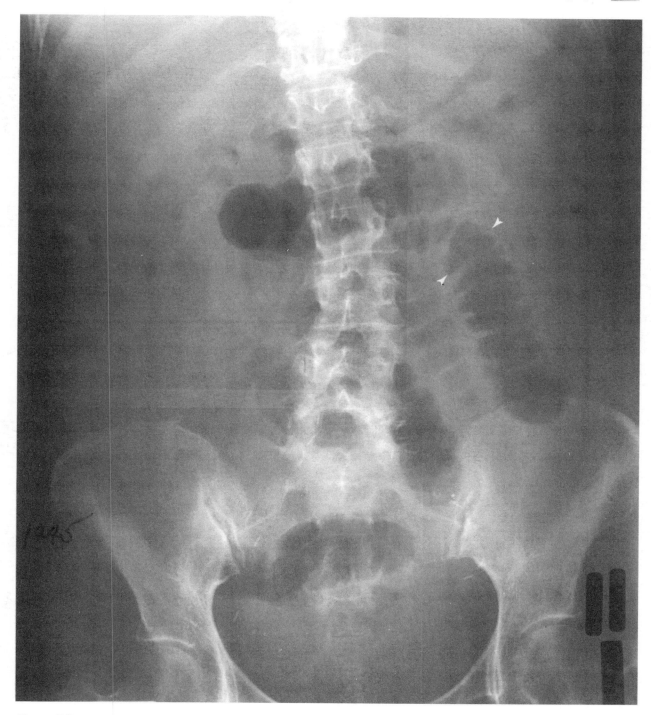

Figure 5-2.

Physical Exam

An essential portion of the physical exam is the presence of high-pitched, "tinkling" bowel sounds, as intestinal contents attempt to squeeze through a narrowed lumen. Abdominal distension is often seen as a late finding, as small bowel loops fill with gas and fluid. The abdomen may be tympanitic to percussion due to gaseous distension.

Diagnostic Evaluation

The first test to order in suspected small bowel obstruction is the acute abdominal series, which consists of three films: an upright chest x-ray, an upright KUB and a supine KUB (Figures 5-1, 5-2). The difference between a KUB and an abdominal plain film is the position of the film over the abdomen. The KUB, as its name implies, is a radiograph that includes the kidneys, ureters, and bladder. The abdominal plain film visualizes the top of the diaphragm and does not include as much of the lower abdomen as the KUB, usually only to the level of the iliac crests. Bowel obstruction may also be diagnosed with a CT of the abdomen in patients who present with abdominal pain (Figure 5-3). CT often demonstrates the site of obstruction as well as inflammation or neoplastic involvement. Oral contrast is preferable, but not absolutely necessary. A small bowel series with oral contrast is often performed in an attempt to elucidate the point of obstruction, but these exams often take several hours due to the delayed transit time through the obstructed intestine and are of limited value.

Radiologic Findings

The acute abdominal series often has air-fluid levels on the upright KUB (Figure 5-1) and dilated loops of small bowel on the supine KUB (Figure 5-2). Small bowel is differentiated from colon by its valvulae conniventes or plica circulares. These are the transverse folds that completely encircle the small bowel as opposed to the colonic haustra, which only cover about half the transverse distance across a given segment of colon. The exclusion of free gas under the diaphragms on the chest radiograph is important, because if it is present it indicates a perforated viscus. If biliary gas is seen centrally within the liver, it is usually the result of prior biliary surgery; although gallstone ileus is also a rare consideration. If portal venous gas is seen at the periphery of the liver, ischemic bowel should be high on the differential diagnosis. The presence of ascites increases the concern for bowel perforation, underlying malignancy, or peritonitis.

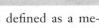

CROHN'S DISEASE

Anatomy

Crohn's disease is a form of chronic inflammatory bowel disease that classically affects the terminal ileum. It is not limited to this area, however; and may affect any portion of the gastrointestinal tract from the oropharynx to the rectum. Classically it occurs in "skip lesions" where there are portions of affected bowel separated by segments of normal bowel. This is in contrast to ulcerative colitis, the other form of inflammatory bowel disease, which affects the colon from the rectum proximally in a continuous fashion.

Etiology

Crohn's disease is considered idiopathic in etiology. Some pathologists speculate that it is an autoimmune-type of disorder, which is aggravated by stress, excessive caffeine intake and smoking cessation. Other theories suggest that it is a chronic infectious process, from a yet undiscovered pathogen.

Pathogenesis

Crohn's disease causes deep ulceration of the intestine that involves the mucosa and lamina propria. Aphthous and linear ulcers are seen grossly and non-caseating granulomas, fissures, and fistulae are seen on microscopic examination of the affected bowel. Crypt abscesses with neutrophils aggregated within mucosal crypt lumens are highly associated with the disease.

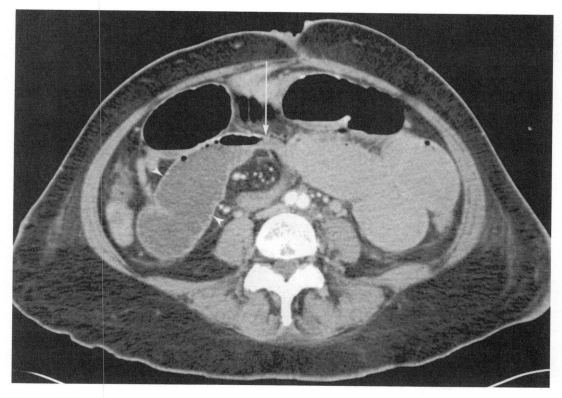

Figure 5-3. Small bowel obstruction. CT appearance of a small bowel obstruction with dilated loops of small bowel filled with gas and fluid. There is a transition point (white arrow) where the bowel narrows and is decompressed distally. This is the point of obstruction and is due to adhesions. (Used with permission of Cedars-Sinai Medical Center, Los Angeles, California.)

Epidemiology

Incidence is approximately 3 per 100,000 in the United States and there is some genetic predisposition, with approximately 15% of patients having a first-degree relative with inflammatory bowel disease. It is more common in Caucasians and affects women more than men in a 1.5 to 1 distribution. The peak age of onset is between 15 and 25, but may occur later in life.

History

Chronic diarrhea that is often blood-tinged, fever, abdominal pain, and anorexia are the most common presenting symptoms. Weight loss, fistulae, and intestinal obstruction commonly occur at some time during the course of the disease.

Extraintestinal manifestations including migratory polyarthritis, sacroiliitis, ankylosing spondylitis, tendency toward gallstone and renal calculus formation, and erythema nodosum all occur, but are not common. There is also an association with sclerosing cholangitis.

Physical Exam

The abdominal exam is less significant than expected. Often patients have only mild abdominal tenderness. Fistulae may be seen upon inspection of the perineum. Rectal exam occasionally demonstrates hemepositive stool.

Diagnostic Evaluation

Generally, an upper gastrointestinal exam with a small-bowel contrast series is the first radiologic test if Crohn's disease is suspected. Laboratory evaluation includes elevated erythrocyte sedimentation rate (ESR), hemoglobin level to determine if anemia is present, and albumin level in severe cases where weight loss has

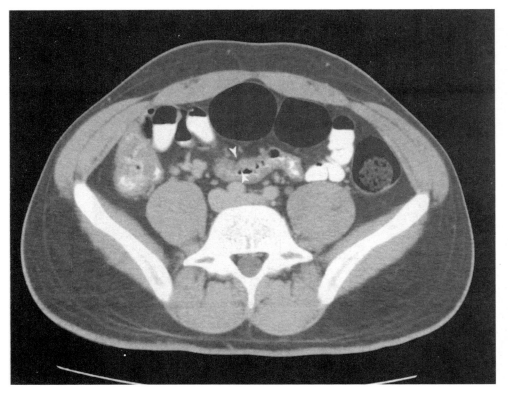

Figure 5-4. Crohn's disease. 22 year-old male patient with inflammation of the terminal ileum consistent with Crohn's disease. Oral contrast consisting of dilute Gastrografin is given one hour prior to the scan and helps to distinguish loops of bowel from lymph nodes, vessels, and other abdominal structures. (Used with permission of Cedars-Sinai Medical Center, Los Angeles, California.)

occurred. Colonoscopy with ileoscopy and biopsy can confirm a suspected diagnosis.

Radiologic Findings

On CT scan, thickening of the wall of the terminal ileum raises suspicion for the diagnosis (Figure 5-4). Inflammation of the adjacent mesenteric fat, abscesses, and fistulae often occur in more severe cases. On barium upper GI and small bowel series examinations, areas of thickened mucosa are seen, classically on the mesenteric side of the bowel. Skip lesions denote areas of affected bowel interspersed between normal-appearing mucosa. Deep, "rose-thorn" ulcerations in the small bowel are often seen (Figure 5-5). Strictures and fistulae to other loops of bowel, bladder, vagina, or skin surface are highly specific for Crohn's disease. Generally, plain radiographs are not helpful in the initial diagnosis, but may be useful in follow-up if small bowel obstruction is suspected, and in diagnosing extraintestinal manifestations such as sacroiliitis and spondylitis.

◆ KEY POINTS ◆

1. Crohn's disease is a form of chronic inflammatory bowel disease that classically affects the terminal ileum, but may also involve any portion of the GI tract.

2. Chronic diarrhea, fever, abdominal pain, and anorexia are the most common presenting symptoms.

3. On barium examination, areas of thickened mucosa with skip lesions, "rose-thorn" ulcerations, strictures, and fistulae are common findings.

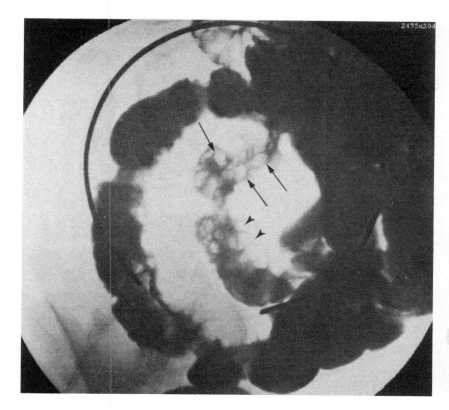

Figure 5-5. Crohn's disease. Spot film from a fluoroscopic small bowel examination, which demonstrates a narrowed loop of ileum with a "cobblestone" appearance of the mucosa (arrows) and deep "rose thorn" ulcers (arrowheads)—findings associated with Crohn's disease. (Used with permission of Cedars-Sinai Medical Center, Los Angeles, California.)

PANCREATITIS

Anatomy

The pancreas is a retroperitoneal structure, which is anatomically divided into four portions: the head, which includes the uncinate process; neck; body; and tail. Its physiologic purpose is to produce and secrete digestive enzymes, insulin, glucagon and several other enzymes important for digestion and metabolism.

Etiology

Acute pancreatitis occurs as a result of many causes, but is most commonly associated with ethanol abuse and choledocholithiasis. Other causes include trauma, Mycoplasma or Coxsackie virus infection, pancreatic neoplasm, hypercalcemia, hyperlipidemia, and certain medications including thiazide diuretics, tetracycline, and sulfonamides. Causes of chronic pancreatitis are usually related to alcohol use and biliary tract disease, and, less commonly, hyperlipidemia.

Pathogenesis

The underlying causes are varied but the mechanism of acute pancreatitis is an inflammatory process that cascades due to auto-digestion of the gland from the enzymes it produces. Chronic pancreatitis, which is usually associated with chronic alcohol use, results in progressive functional destruction of the gland with exocrine and endocrine deficiencies.

Epidemiology

The approximate incidence of pancreatitis is 10 to 20 per 100,000 in the United States. Men and women are generally equally affected. The peak age of incidence is between ages 30 and 40, which is mostly related to alcohol consumption. There is not usually a genetic association, although there is a rare autosomal dominant form of inherited predisposition to pancreatitis.

History

Patients typically present with complaints of midepigastric abdominal pain that may radiate through to the

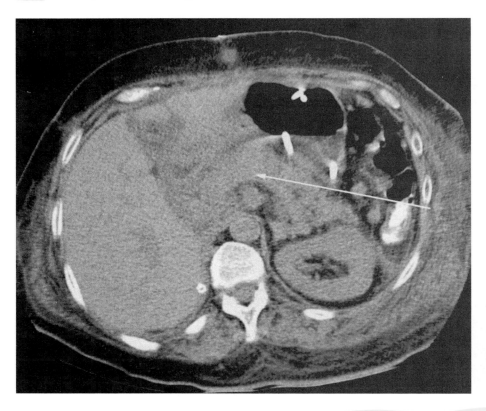

Figure 5-6. Acute pancreatitis. CT appearance of acute pancreatitis with edema of the pancreas and inflammatory changes or "stranding" of the peripancreatic fat. (Used with permission of Cedars-Sinai Medical Center, Los Angeles, California.)

back. Nausea, vomiting, and fever are common symptoms. Past medical history may include symptomatology of cholelithiasis, including intermittent bouts of postprandial right upper quadrant pain and steatorrhea.

Physical Exam

Fever, jaundice, abdominal tenderness and absent or diminished bowel sounds are common physical findings. Abdominal distension may occur secondary to a paralytic ileus. More severe cases may have hypotension, tachycardia, and shock physiology. Grey Turner's sign with flank discoloration or Cullen's sign with umbilical discoloration are also classic physical findings seen in some cases.

Diagnostic Evaluation

Laboratory evaluation includes a serum lipase level in suspected cases. An elevated lipase level is more specific for pancreatitis than a serum amylase level because many other pathologic conditions such as esophageal rupture, intestinal obstruction, and perforated peptic ulcer may present with an elevated amylase level and similar symptoms. Ranson's criteria, which predict prognosis in pancreatitis, include initial labs of: white

blood cell (WBC) count greater than 16,000, serum glucose greater than 200, serum LDH (lactate dehydrogenase) greater than 350, and serumglutámic-oxaloacetic transaminase (SGOT) greater than 250.

Pancreatitis is commonly considered a clinical diagnosis, but imaging is useful, especially in potential surgical cases with pseudocyst or abscess. Radiographic evaluation usually begins with an acute abdominal series including flat and upright KUB and upright AP chest radiograph. Ultrasound of the abdomen is helpful if the pancreas can be visualized, but it is often obscured by overlying bowel gas. If pancreatitis is high on the differential diagnosis, a CT scan of the abdomen with contrast may confirm the diagnosis. Follow-up CT scans may be performed if there is concern for pseudocyst or abscess formation.

Radiologic Findings

The acute abdominal series often demonstrates a diffuse paralytic ileus pattern. A "sentinel loop" of small bowel in the left upper quadrant represents a focal ileus adjacent to the area of pancreatic inflammation. The "colon cutoff sign" is also strongly associated with pancreatitis and appears as a distended, gas-filled,

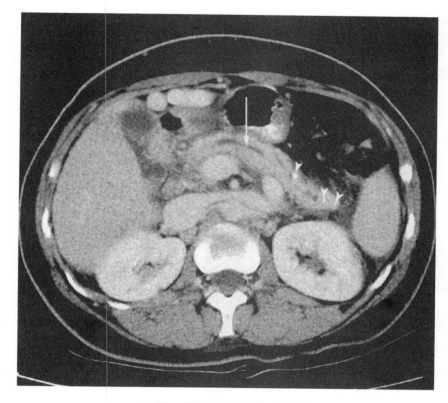

Figure 5-7. Chronic pancreatitis. Early contrast phase of abdominal CT that demonstrates dilated pancreatic duct (white arrow), pancreatic calcifications (arrowheads), and subtle pancreatic inflammation. (Used with permission of Cedars-Sinai Medical Center, Los Angeles, California.)

transverse colon with no colonic gas seen distal to the splenic flexure. A left pleural effusion is a relatively common finding. Calcified gallstones seen on plain radiographs may give an indication as to the cause of pancreatitis.

Ultrasound frequently reveals an edematous, enlarged pancreas, sometimes with dilatation of the pancreatic duct. Gallstones are easily visualized within the gallbladder on ultrasound; however, the distal body and tail of the pancreas are often poorly visualized by ultrasound and inflammation in these areas can be missed.

CT scan can provide a definitive diagnosis of pancreatitis with findings of pancreatic edema, peripancreatic fat inflammation and fluid (Figure 5-6), and pancreatic or common bile duct dilatation (Figure 5-7). Intravenous iodine-based contrast is of value in determining the degree of pancreatic necrosis, which correlates strongly with morbidity. Follow-up CT scans are useful for diagnosing the complications of pancreatitis such as pseudocyst and abscess formation. Chronic pancreatitis is associated with atrophy of the gland, scattered calcifications, and pancreatic duct dilatation.

◆ KEY POINTS ◆

1. Acute pancreatitis may occur as a result of many causes, but is most commonly associated with ethanol intoxication and choledocholithiasis.

2. Patients typically present with complaints of midepigastric abdominal pain that radiates through to the back, nausea, vomiting, and fever.

3. Diagnostic evaluation should include a serum lipase level and an acute abdominal series.

4. A paralytic ileus pattern, "sentinel loop," and "colon cutoff sign" are common radiographic findings associated with pancreatitis.

5. Ultrasound may be useful in some cases if pancreatic edema is demonstrated, but is often nonspecific.

6. CT scan of the abdomen with intravenous contrast frequently provides a definitive diagnosis of pancreatitis with findings of pancreatic edema, peripancreatic fat inflammation and fluid, and pancreatic or common bile duct dilatation.

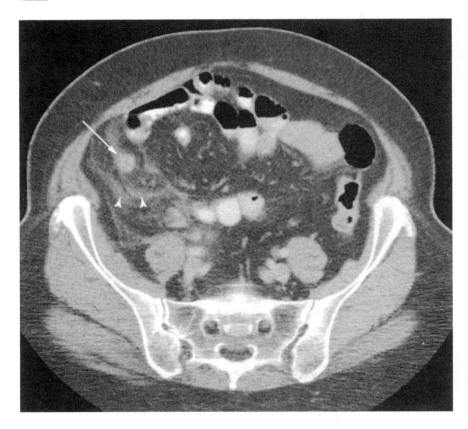

Figure 5-8. Acute appendicitis. CT of the abdomen demonstrates a dilated, thick-walled appendix seen in cross-section (arrow) with adjacent inflammation of the periappendiceal fat (arrowheads). (Used with permission of Cedars-Sinai Medical Center, Los Angeles, California.)

APPENDICITIS

Anatomy

The appendix is a vestigial structure located at the tip of the cecum in the right lower quadrant of the abdomen. Normally it measures less than 5 mm in diameter and has a wall thickness less than 3 mm. It has many anatomic variants in its position and length. It may be closely apposed to the posterior wall of the cecum (retrocecal), adjacent to the right psoas muscle, or in the pelvis.

Etiology

The most common cause of appendicitis is obstruction of the appendiceal lumen, usually by an appendicolith. Other uncommon causes include obstruction by lymphoid tissue hypertrophy or neoplasm, often carcinoid tumor.

Pathogenesis

Luminal obstruction leads to bacterial overgrowth and subsequent inflammation. Secondarily there is venous obstruction, ischemia and necrosis. Some cases may progress to appendiceal rupture and peritoneal infection.

Epidemiology

Appendicitis is the most common acute surgical condition and will affect approximately 7% of all people over the course of a lifetime. The incidence is estimated at 10 to 20 per 100,000 in the United States. There is a slight predominance for occurrence of appendicitis in men, especially in adolescents and young adults; however, it may occur at any age.

History

Patients present first with anorexia, then with abdominal pain that classically begins in the periumbilical area and then gradually moves to McBurney's point, which is located at two-thirds the distance from the umbilicus to the right anterior superior iliac spine. Vomiting may occur later as pain increases in right lower quadrant.

Physical Exam

Rebound tenderness in the right lower quadrant and guarding are classic physical findings of acute appendicitis. Other signs include the psoas sign, which is pain in the deep upper pelvis during extension of a flexed right

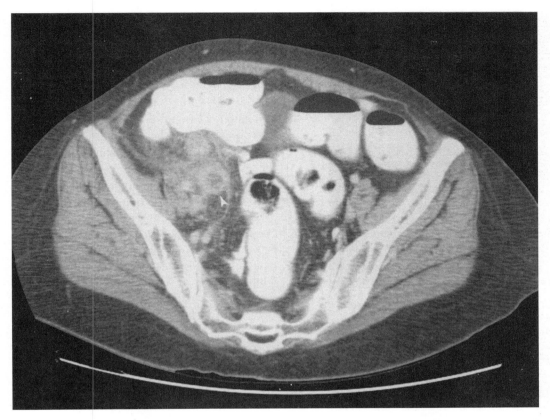

Figure 5-9. Acute appendicitis. CT with dilute oral contrast demonstrates non-filling of a markedly dilated appendix and inflammation of the periappendiceal fat. (Used with permission of Cedars-Sinai Medical Center, Los Angeles, California.)

thigh against examiner resistance. The obturator sign is pain during internal rotation of a flexed right thigh against examiner resistance. A retrocecal appendix may give right flank tenderness to palpation, and an appendix located deep within the pelvis may give local and suprapubic tenderness on rectal exam. Low-grade fever is common at presentation and may increase as symptoms progress. High fevers with peritoneal signs are associated with appendiceal rupture. Often just after the appendix ruptures, patients will notice a sudden decrease in pain.

Diagnostic Evaluation

Appendicitis remains largely a clinical diagnosis. History and physical exam point to the diagnosis and the labs and radiographs will either confirm or point toward another cause of the symptoms. Laboratory evaluation usually demonstrates elevated WBC count (10,000 to 20,000) with a left shift (polymorphonuclear cells (PMNs) >75%

on differential). 25% of patients will have either hematuria or evidence of white blood cells in the urine.

Radiologic evaluation may be very useful in cases of intermediate suspicion based on history and physical. Generally, plain radiographs are useful as an initial screening study for abdominal pain, but normal findings should not delay the diagnosis if there are classical findings on the history and physical. Both ultrasound (performed preferentially in children and pregnant women) and CT in all other patients are highly accurate studies in diagnosing acute appendicitis. Gastrografin enemas are nonspecific and should not be performed.

Radiologic Findings

On CT scan the appendix is often dilated, greater than 6 mm in transverse diameter. There is often inflammation of the fat surrounding the appendix (Figure 5-8). Adjacent free fluid or a fluid-filled mass

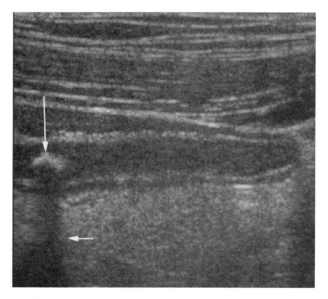

Figure 5-10. Acute appendicitis. Ultrasound of the right lower quadrant demonstrates a non-compressible, thick-walled appendix and an echogenic, shadowing (small arrow) appendicolith (large arrow). (Used with permission of Cedars-Sinai Medical Center, Los Angeles, California.)

may indicate appendiceal perforation. Occasionally, a calcified appendicolith is present within the lumen of the appendix. If rectal contrast has been given, nonfilling of the appendix suggests luminal obstruction and a positive diagnosis (Figure 5-9). If the appendix completely fills with contrast, then appendicitis is virtually excluded.

US examination commonly reveals a dilated, non-compressible tubular structure in the right lower quadrant representing the appendix (Figure 5-10). This is often seen over the point of maximal tenderness. Occasionally, a calcified appendicolith is seen as a highly echogenic structure with posterior shadowing in the proximal portion of the appendix. Adjacent inflammation and fluid may be seen but are sometimes obscured by overlying bowel gas.

◆ KEY POINTS ◆

1. The most common cause of appendicitis is obstruction of the appendiceal lumen, usually by an appendicolith.

2. Appendicitis is the most common acute surgical condition and it will affect approximately 7% of all people over the course of a lifetime.

3. Patients present with anorexia and abdominal pain that begins in the periumbilical area, then moves to McBurney's point.

4. Rebound tenderness and guarding in the right lower quadrant are classic physical findings of appendicitis. Other signs include the psoas sign and the obturator sign.

5. Ultrasound examination commonly reveals a dilated, tender, non-compressible tubular structure in the right lower quadrant.

6. On CT scan, stranding of the periappendiceal fat, a dilated appendix greater than 6 mm and an appendicolith are highly specific findings.

DIVERTICULITIS

Anatomy

Colonic diverticula are outpouchings of the mucosa and submucosa through the muscularis layer. They occur at areas of weakness in the muscularis that align along the points where nutrient vessels pierce the muscularis. Diverticula are most commonly located in the sigmoid colon, may occasionally be seen in the ascending, transverse, and descending portions of the colon, and do not occur in the rectum.

Etiology

The formation of diverticula is thought to occur due to lack of fiber in the diet. High fiber intake allows faster transit through the colon and the formation of softer stool that is easily passed. Slow transit through the colon, hard stool, and higher than normal pressures in the sigmoid colon force the mucosa and submucosa out through the weak areas in the muscularis layer, leading to diverticulosis.

Pathogenesis

Diverticulitis occurs when diverticula become obstructed and there is subsequent overgrowth of bacteria within the outpouching. The infected diverticulum may

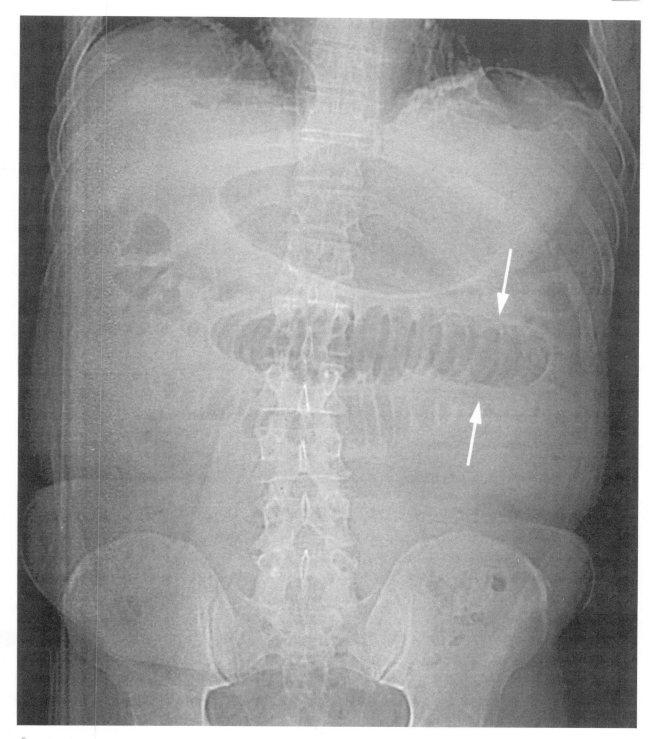

Figure 5-11. KUB demonstrating dilated loops of small bowel in a pattern of obstruction or ileus. The patient presented with fever, elevated WBC count, and left lower quadrant pain and was diagnosed with diverticulitis on CT scan. (Used with permission of Cedars-Sinai Medical Center, Los Angeles, California.)

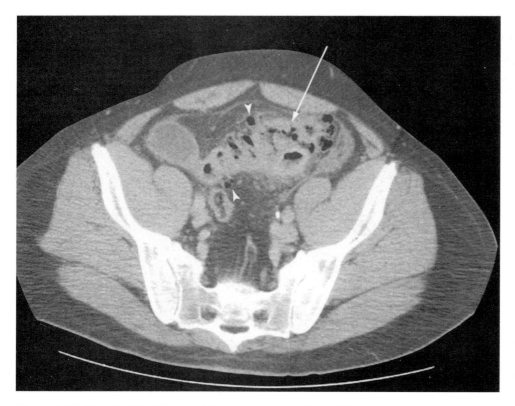

Figure 5-12. Diverticulitis. CT scan of the same patient in Figure 5-11 demonstrates a thick-walled sigmoid colon with inflammation of the adjacent fat (white arrow) and multiple diverticula (white arrowheads). (Used with permission of Cedars-Sinai Medical Center, Los Angeles, California.)

have microperforation, causing localized inflammation or frank perforation leading to abscess formation.

Epidemiology

Incidence increases with age and is estimated at 3000 per 100,000 in the United States. It is rare before age 40 and affects men and women equally. There is no genetic predisposition, but it is more common in Western society, likely due to low fiber diet. Patients with prior history of diverticulitis are at increased risk of developing recurrent episodes.

History

Patients with diverticulosis may be asymptomatic or may have intermittent bouts of bleeding. Often, diverticula are found incidentally at screening colonoscopy. About 25% of patients with diverticulosis will develop diverticulitis at some point in their life. They often present with left lower quadrant pain, low-grade fever and anorexia, nausea and vomiting.

Physical Exam

The most common physical findings of diverticulitis are left lower quadrant rebound tenderness, guarding, and palpable mass. Diffuse peritoneal signs such as non-localized rebound tenderness or guarding are suggestive of perforation and peritonitis. Bowel sounds may be diminished if there is paralytic ileus.

Diagnostic Evaluation

Radiographs are usually nonspecific but may demonstrate evidence of obstruction or ileus (Figure 5-11). CT scan of the abdomen combined with laboratory evaluation of WBC count are specific for the diagnosis.

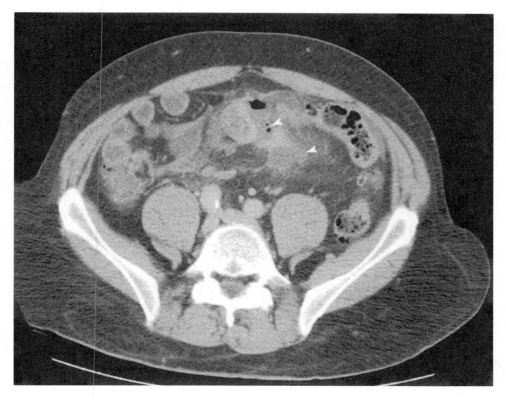

Figure 5-13. Diverticulitis. CT scan reveals inflammation of the pericolonic fat and a small collection of extraluminal gas and fluid representing a microperforation from diverticulitis. (Used with permission of Cedars-Sinai Medical Center, Los Angeles, California.)

A CT of the abdomen is useful in determining if there is associated abscess formation and safe access for drainage catheter placement.

Radiologic Findings

The CT scan frequently demonstrates colonic wall thickening, inflammation of the adjacent mesenteric fat (Figure 5-12), and occasionally small pockets of extraluminal gas suggesting microperforation (Figure 5-13). Diverticula are present in the involved segment of colon. Abscess formation often occurs in the evolution of an episode of diverticulitis. Oral and/or rectal contrast given prior to the exam may help in the diagnosis but are not absolutely necessary. A perforated colonic carcinoma may mimic diverticulitis, but more pronounced focal wall thickening or a focal mass is often present.

◆ KEY POINTS ◆

1. Colonic diverticula are outpouchings of the mucosa and submucosa through the muscularis layer, thought to occur due to lack of fiber in the diet.

2. Diverticulitis occurs when diverticula become obstructed and there is subsequent overgrowth of bacteria.

3. The most common physical findings of diverticulitis are left lower quadrant rebound tenderness, guarding, and palpable mass.

4. CT findings include colonic wall thickening, inflammation of the adjacent mesenteric fat, and small pockets of extraluminal gas and fluid.

6

Urologic Imaging

NEPHROLITHIASIS

Anatomy

Renal calculi occur throughout the urinary tract and may be seen incidentally on plain films overlying the renal shadow, in the ureter, or in the bladder. They initially form in the proximal urinary tract and may move distally, sometimes passing during urination. The three most common points where they become obstructed are the ureteropelvic junction (UPJ), the point where the ureter crosses over the iliac vessels, and the ureterovesicular junction (UVJ) (Figure 6-1).

Etiology

Renal stones are generally of four basic types:

1. Calcium oxalate or calcium phosphate (75%);
2. Struvite (magnesium ammonium phosphate) (approximately 15%), which are associated with alkalinized urine and infections;
3. Uric acid (8%) associated with gout and multiple myeloma;
4. Cystine (2%) stones associated with cystinuria.

A small percentage (<1%) of stones also occur as precipitates of medications. One of these medications is indinavir, a common HIV protease inhibitor. The stones from indinavir are notable because, unlike the other types of stones listed above, they are non-opaque and are not visible on a noncontrast CT.

Pathogenesis

Stones form when urine becomes supersaturated with crystals, which begin to precipitate. Precipitation may be increased or decreased depending on the pH of the urine and the type of crystal being formed.

Epidemiology

Patients usually present between the ages of 30 and 50. Predisposing conditions include Crohn's disease, calyceal

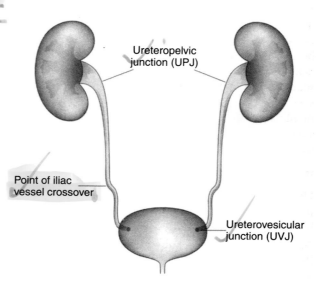

Figure 6-1. Common points of ureteral obstruction from calculi. (Illustration by Electronic Illustrators Group.)

diverticula, hypercalcemia, and renal tubular acidosis. Calcium stones are more common in men at a 3:1 ratio with women. Struvite stones are slightly more common in women. Approximately 1 in 10 people will have renal stones at some point during their lifetime.

History

Patients with nephrolithiasis often present with flank pain known as "renal colic" that waxes and wanes as the ureter contracts against the stone. The pain may radiate to the bladder area or groin.

Physical Examination

On exam, there is pain at the costovertebral angle on the affected side. Some patients have chills and fever if there is an associated infection. Hematuria is common; however, it may be microscopic rather than gross.

Diagnostic Evaluation

An elevated white blood cell count with predominant granulocytes is common on laboratory evaluation. Plain films of the abdomen may demonstrate a calcification in 80–90% of patients, but small stones in the pelvis are difficult to distinguish from phleboliths. Urate calculi are radiolucent on plain radiographs. Historically, the intravenous pyelogram (IVP) was the diagnostic test of choice to evaluate for obstruction and determine the size and location of calculi. The CT urogram without contrast has replaced the IVP. It is performed much faster, avoids the risks of iodinated contrast, and has a decreased radiation dose to the patient compared to an IVP. A decreased radiation dose is especially important to patients of childbearing age, because a significant amount of radiation is delivered to the pelvis and gonads during an IVP. Ultrasound of the kidneys also shows calcifications as echodensities with posterior shadowing. Hydronephrosis is commonly visualized with ultrasound if there is an obstructing stone; however, ultrasound is inherently neither as sensitive nor specific as CT in diagnosing ureteral obstruction.

Radiographic Findings

Historically, the first imaging study performed for suspected nephrolithiasis has been the kidneys, ureter, and bladder radiograph (KUB) to evaluate for calcifications. Approximately 80 to 90% of urinary tract calculi will appear radiodense on plain radiographs. Urate crystals are not well visualized on plain radiographs. Some clinicians order an IVP to confirm a suspected calcification seen on plain radiographs. Contrast material concentrates in

the kidneys and provides information about the size of the kidneys and their relative function. The affected kidney may appear larger with a persistent nephrogram. There is delayed opacification of the collecting system on the affected side. A urinary tract calculus appears as a filling defect in the collecting system or ureter. Hydronephrosis and/or hydroureter may be present depending on the level of obstruction.

The noncontrast CT urogram has replaced the KUB and IVP as the preferred method of imaging in suspected nephrolithiasis. The risks of contrast are avoided, there is a reduced radiation dose, and in most cases the exam can be performed and interpreted in much less time. Nearly all renal calculi will appear as high attenuation on CT, with the exception of indinavir precipitates. The main finding in acute urolithiasis on CT is a calcification in the affected collecting system (Fig 6-2a, b), ureter or in the bladder. Mild hydronephrosis often persists after the stone has already passed. Other findings that may support the diagnosis include inflammation and fluid in the perinephric fat caused by edema and/or urine released from a ruptured fornix. Large stones in the proximal ureter rarely pass, and small stones in the distal ureter commonly pass with time.

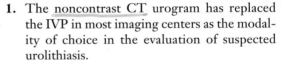

◆ KEY POINTS ◆

1. The noncontrast CT urogram has replaced the IVP in most imaging centers as the modality of choice in the evaluation of suspected urolithiasis.

2. The diagnosis of urolithiasis is made with CT when an obstructing stone is visualized and associated with dilatation of the proximal ureter and/or collecting system.

3. Calcifications are seen at the ureteropelvic junction, the point where the ureter crosses over the iliac vessels, and at the ureterovesicular junction.

TESTICULAR TORSION

Anatomy

The testes are suspended within the scrotum by the spermatic cords. The spermatic cords contain the ductus deferens and the blood vessels, nerves, and lymphatics for the testes. The testes are covered by the dense,

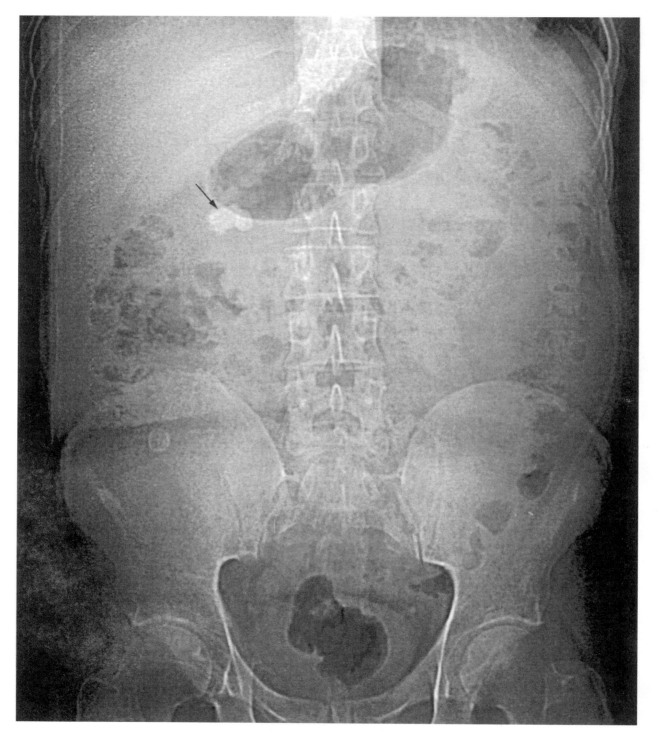

Figure 6-2a. Urolithiasis. KUB demonstrates a large right renal calcification. (Used with permission of Cedars-Sinai Medical Center, Los Angeles, California.)

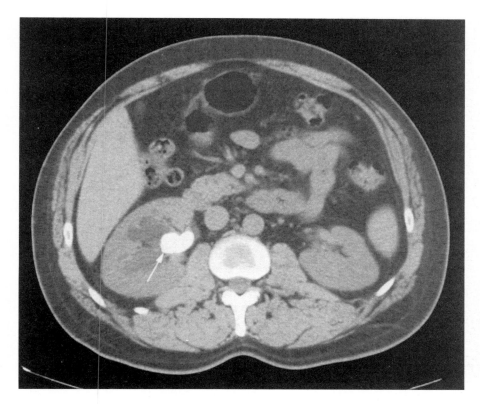

Figure 6-2b. Urolithiasis. CT of the same patient in Figure 6-2a with right renal collecting system calculus. (Used with permission of Cedars-Sinai Medical Center, Los Angeles, California.)

fibrous tunica albuginea, which is partially covered by the visceral and parietal layers of the tunica vaginalis. The testes are normally fixed in place within the scrotum by the gubernaculum.

Etiology

Testicular torsion is a true radiographic emergency. It is caused by rotation of the testis and spermatic cord causing venous and eventually arterial occlusion and subsequent infarction of the affected testis. Trauma or strenuous physical exertion are often the cause. The bell-clapper deformity is a congenital anatomic variant in which there is congenital absence of the gubernaculum, the posterior attachment of the tunica vaginalis to the scrotum. With a bell-clapper deformity the testis is only loosely connected to the scrotum and is able to move freely within the scrotal sac and twist (torse) around the axis of the blood vessels (Figure 6-3). The bell-clapper variant is bilateral in 50 to 80% of cases.

Epidemiology

Torsion presents at any age, but most commonly occurs in two peaks, neonates and in the second decade.

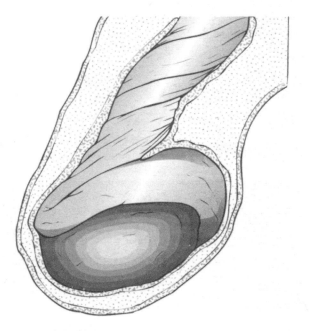

Figure 6-3. Testicular torsion due to bell-clapper deformity. (Used with permission from Karp SJ, Morris JPG, Soybel DI. Blueprints in Surgery, 2nd Ed. Malden: Blackwell Science, Inc., 2001:53.)

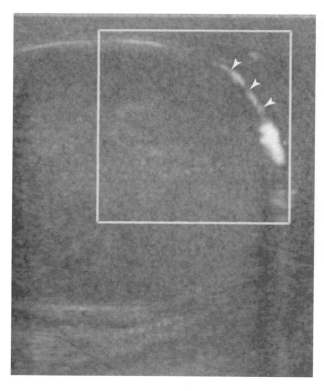

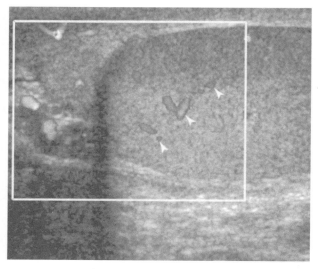

Figure 6-4b. Normal Doppler flow ultrasound in left testis of the same patient as 6-4a. Arrowheads show areas of blood flow. (Used with permission of Cedars-Sinai Medical Center, Los Angeles, California.)

Figure 6-4a. Testicular torsion. Ultrasound of the testis with Doppler flow imaging demonstrates lack of blood flow within the torsed right testis. There is flow peripherally. (Used with permission of Cedars-Sinai Medical Center, Los Angeles, California.)

History

Patients usually present with sudden onset of testicular pain, increasing in severity as ischemia progresses.

Physical Examination

On exam, the affected testis is tender, enlarged, and may be edematous, and erythematous. It is often located high in the scrotum, sometimes oriented with the long axis horizontal rather than the normal vertical position. There may be an absent cremasteric reflex, which is the normal retraction of the scrotum and testis when the ipsilateral inner thigh is lightly scratched. The presentation often mimics epididymo-orchitis and an incarcerated inguinal hernia, which are the two major differential diagnostic considerations. Other differential diagnoses include traumatic hematoma, varicocele, hydrocele, scrotal abscess, and testicular tumor.

Diagnostic Evaluation

Ultrasonography with Doppler and nuclear scintigraphy are two commonly used imaging modalities; however ultrasound can be performed more rapidly and is the test of

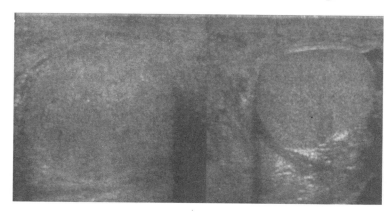

Figure 6-4c. Testicular torsion. Side-by-side comparison with grayscale ultrasound reveals heterogeneous echotexture of the torsed right testis compared to the normal left testis. The patient had the acute onset of pain after falling from a skateboard. (Used with permission of Cedars-Sinai Medical Center, Los Angeles, California.)

choice. Other diagnoses which may mimic torsion such as epididymitis and orchitis can be diagnosed with ultrasound as well. Rapid diagnosis and treatment of testicular torsion is essential, because the salvage rate drops off quickly after 6 hours. At 12 hours, the salvage rate is approximately 20%. At 24 hours the chance of salvage is virtually zero.

Radiologic Findings

Ultrasound with color-flow Doppler reveals absent or decreased blood flow (Figure 6-4a, b) in the affected testis during the acute period (<6 hrs). Comparison is made to the unaffected side. During the acute period, testicular torsion can be distinguished from epididymo-orchitis, which has increased blood flow due to the inflammatory process. Incarcerated inguinal hernia will have normal blood flow to the testis, and ultrasound may reveal the contents of the hernia. During the late period (>24 hours), grayscale ultrasound imaging shows heterogeneity of the affected testis (Figure 6-4c) and absent blood flow within the testis itself. There may be increased blood flow with color-flow Doppler around the periphery of the testis as inflammation increases.

Nuclear scintigraphy may be used as an adjunct to testicular ultrasound imaging. It is not used in children, <2 years old because the testes are too small to be identified by the gamma cameras. The finding of a unilateral "cold" or photopenic testis is positive for testicular torsion. Another sign used to identify testicular torsion on nuclear imaging is the "ring sign." With this finding, activity around the testis with a central photopenic zone of no activity signifies inflammation around an ischemic or necrotic testis.

◆ KEY POINTS ◆

1. Testicular torsion is a true radiographic emergency. It is caused by rotation of the testis and spermatic cord causing venous and eventually arterial occlusion and subsequent infarction of the affected testis.
2. The bell-clapper deformity is a risk factor.
3. The two major differential diagnostic considerations presentation are epididymo-orchitis and an incarcerated inguinal hernia.
4. Ultrasound with Doppler color-flow imaging is the test of choice, and reveals absent or decreased blood flow in the affected testis during the acute period (<6 hrs).

7

Obstetric and Gynecologic Imaging

ANATOMY

The adnexal structures, including the ovaries, fallopian tubes, and ovarian vessels, are connected to the uterus by the broad ligament. The fimbriae of the fallopian tubes wrap around the ovaries but are also open to the peritoneal cavity. An ovum released from an ovarian follicle remains free in the peritoneal cavity for a brief amount of time before being swept into the fallopian tube by the fimbriae (Figure 7-1).

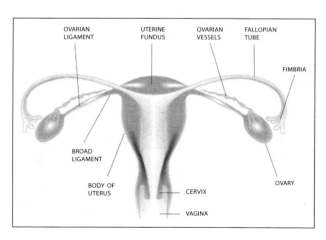

Figure 7-1. Normal anatomy of the female reproductive organs. (Illustration by Shawn Girsberger Graphic Design.)

OVARIAN TORSION

Etiology

Ovarian torsion is a result of rotation of the ovary around its vascular supply. Adnexal mass is usually the cause as the ovarian ligament and the broad ligament cannot support the weight of the mass in normal anatomic position. Common adnexal masses include ovarian neoplasms, polycystic ovary, large ovarian cysts, endometriomas, and dermoid cysts (Figure 7-2).

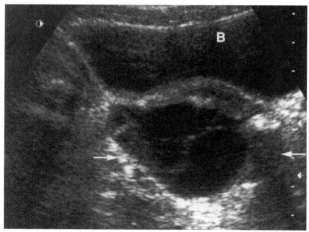

Figure 7-2. Dermoid cyst. Ultrasound of the pelvis demonstrates a complex cystic mass in the adnexa, which was found to be a dermoid cyst. (Used with permission of Cedars-Sinai Medical Center, Los Angeles, California.)

Pathogenesis

When ovarian torsion occurs, venous return is obstructed and the ovary becomes edematous. The edema adds to the weight and volume of the ovary, often leading to further torsion. The ovary becomes ischemic due to the reduced flow of arterial blood, especially in small and medium-sized vessels.

Epidemiology

Ovarian torsion occurs in women of any age, but is most common in childhood and adolescence. In childhood, the cause is usually a large dermoid tumor (teratoma), which is the most common ovarian tumor in preadolescent women. In young adult women, large ovarian cysts are the most common cause of torsion. In postmenopausal women, ovarian adenocarcinoma is the most common cause.

History

Women often present to the emergency room complaining of extreme, acute-onset pelvic pain. The acute nature of the pain relates to the fact that a slow-growing mass may not cause pain, but when it acts as a lead point for torsion, the subsequent ischemia to the affected ovary is acutely painful.

Physical Exam

With ovarian torsion, there is often deep pain to palpation on the affected side of the pelvis and often generalized pelvic pain. On physical exam, ovarian torsion may mimic appendicitis, with right lower quadrant tenderness, or diverticulitis, with left lower quadrant tenderness. Palpation for adnexal masses during the pelvic exam is important, as they are frequently an underlying cause of ovarian torsion. Vaginal bleeding is not commonly associated with torsion.

Diagnostic Evaluation

The imaging study of choice in the evaluation of acute pelvic pain and/or suspected pelvic mass is ultrasound. The test can be performed quickly and easily from the emergency room without need for preparation. Transvaginal ultrasound provides detailed anatomy of the uterus and adnexae. If ovarian torsion is suspected, the diagnosis should be made within four hours, in order to save the ovary from infarction. Doppler imaging should be a part of the exam to evaluate the blood flow to the affected ovary. Alternatively, MRI of the pelvis without contrast can be done, but may take up to one hour to perform, and there must be no contraindications to MR imaging such

TABLE 7-1
Differential Diagnosis of Acute Pelvic Pain
Ruptured ovarian follicle (most common)
Endometriosis
Pelvic inflammatory disease (PID)
Tubo-ovarian abscess
Ectopic pregnancy
Ovarian torsion
Non-gynecologic causes: Appendicitis
Diverticulitis

as the presence of a pacemaker, intracranial aneurysm clips, or intraorbital metallic foreign bodies.

Lab tests should be performed to exclude pregnancy as a cause of the pelvic pain. Other tests including complete blood count (CBC) and white blood cell (WBC) count are usually normal with ovarian torsion. This may help in excluding pelvic inflammatory disease, tubo-ovarian abscess, or other infectious/inflammatory causes of pelvic pain from the differential diagnosis (Table 7-1).

Radiologic Findings

An adnexal mass greater than 2.5 cm on the side of the pain is the most common ultrasonographic finding in ovarian torsion (Figure 7-3). This is a nonspecific finding

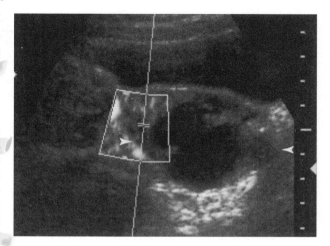

Figure 7-3. Ovarian mass. Ultrasound image of complex cystic and solid ovarian mass. The cursor is placed over an area of blood flow to evaluate for potential torsion. (Used with permission of Cedars-Sinai Medical Center, Los Angeles, California.)

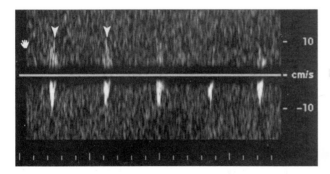

Figure 7-4. Ovarian torsion. Doppler flow tracing demonstrates only arterial blood flow. No venous flow could be identified in the ovary shown in Figure 7-3. (Used with permission of Cedars-Sinai Medical Center, Los Angeles, California.)

and becomes important only when the history, physical, and other findings direct the differential diagnosis towards ovarian torsion. Absence or severe reduction of venous blood flow to the ovary on Doppler color flow imaging (Figure 7-4) is a useful finding, though not diagnostic. However, if venous flow is noted centrally within the ovary, torsion is virtually excluded.

A unilateral enlarged ovary with multiple peripheral cortical follicles and pelvic free fluid are also common, nonspecific findings. The free fluid commonly seen with torsion represents hemorrhage from a necrotic ovary following prolonged arterial occlusion and subsequent ischemia.

◆ KEY POINTS ◆

1. Ovarian torsion is a result of rotation of the ovary around its vascular supply.

2. The most common presenting complaint is acute onset, extreme pelvic pain.

3. The imaging study of choice is ultrasound. + doppler (mass)

4. The diagnosis of ovarian torsion must be made (blood flow) quickly (<4 hours) to save the ovary from infarction.

5. A nonspecific ovarian mass on the side of the pain is the most common ultrasonographic finding in ovarian torsion.

6. Absence or severe reduction of venous blood flow to the ovary on Doppler color flow imaging is a useful finding, though not diagnostic.

7. Venous blood flow centrally within the ovary virtually excludes ovarian torsion.

OVARIAN CARCINOMA

Etiology

Primary ovarian neoplasms are grouped according to the cell-type of origin. The ovary is composed of germ cells, stromal or supporting cells, and epithelial cells that may all give rise to a neoplasm. Epithelial cells that cover the surface of the ovaries give rise to serous or mucinous cystadenocarcinomas, clear cell carcinomas, and endometrioid carcinomas. Germ cells or oocytes are the cell of origin for dysgerminomas, embryonal cell cancers, choriocarcinomas, yolk sac tumors and teratomas (dermoids). Stromal cells give rise to granulosa cell tumors, Sertoli-Leydig cell tumors and fibromas. Other tumors of the ovaries include lymphoma and metastatic tumors commonly from breast, uterine, or gastrointestinal primary malignancies (known as Krukenberg tumors when they metastasize to the ovary).

Epidemiology

Ovarian carcinoma is the fifth leading cause of cancer death in women and comprises 25% of all gynecologic malignancies. The incidence is approximately 20,000 new cases each year with peak incidence at ages 50 to 60. Epithelial cell neoplasms (75% of ovarian tumors) occur in the fifth to eighth decades. Germ cell tumors (15%) occur more often in women aged 12 to 40, although epithelial cell neoplasm is the most common neoplasm in this age group. Stromal tumors make up the remaining 5 to 10% of ovarian tumors.

There is some genetic component to ovarian cancer, with an increased relative risk of 1.5 if there are two first-degree relatives with the disease. The BRCA-1 gene has been implicated in many of these cases with such genetic predisposition.

History

Patients often present to their primary care physician's office with nonspecific complaints of weight loss, abdominal distension, vague abdominal and pelvic discomfort, or the feeling of a pelvic mass. Some patients may present acutely if the mass is large enough to cause torsion and acute pelvic pain. Risk factors that should be elicited during the past medical history are low parity, high-fat high lactose diet, and delayed child-bearing. Oral contraceptive pills statistically have a protective effect.

Physical Exam

Ascites, pelvic mass, and cachexia are late physical examination signs. Unfortunately ovarian neoplasms often present at an advanced stage, often with distant metastases with 65% of patients having metastatic disease at the time of diagnosis. Although CA-125 levels are elevated in most patients with the disease, the test is not specific for ovarian neoplasm and is generally not used as a screening tool, but rather as a way to follow treatment effectiveness in confirmed cases.

Diagnostic Evaluation

Pelvic ultrasound is the imaging modality most often used for suspected ovarian neoplasm. Both transabdominal and transvaginal imaging should be performed. The transabdominal views provide a general survey of the pelvis to evaluate upper pelvic structures, look for lymphadenopathy or peritoneal spread, and to find pelvic free fluid. Transvaginal images define with greater detail the extent of disease in the ovary and adnexa. If torsion is suspected, Doppler imaging should also be performed. The differential diagnosis of an ovarian mass includes both benign and malignant neoplasms, ovarian cysts, torsion, and endometrioma.

Radiologic Findings

The most common ultrasonographic finding with ovarian carcinoma is a unilateral adnexal mass with complex cystic features (Figure 7-5). If the volume of the ovary is

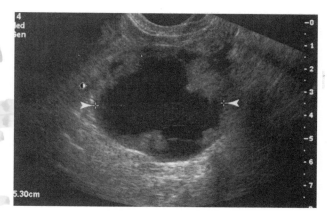

Figure 7-6. Ovarian cystadenocarcinoma. Ultrasound image of mixed cystic and solid ovarian mass. (Used with permission of Cedars-Sinai Medical Center, Los Angeles, California.)

greater than 18 cm³ in premenopausal women, or greater than 8 cm³ in post-menopausal women, it is considered abnormal and suspicious for ovarian neoplasm. Mixed cystic and solid lesions are suggestive of malignancy and occur most commonly with ovarian cystadenocarcinomas (Figure 7-6). Cystic components are identified by lack of internal echoes (appear black on ultrasound) and posterior acoustic enhancement (brightness beyond the cyst).

Other findings that suggest malignancy are listed in Table 7-2:

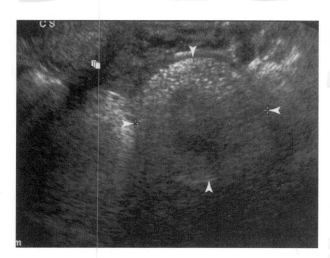

Figure 7-5. Ovarian carcinoma. Ultrasound of large, heterogeneous, echogenic adnexal mass. (Used with permission of Cedars-Sinai Medical Center, Los Angeles, California.)

TABLE 7-2

Ultrasonographic Findings that Suggest Malignant Ovarian Neoplasm

Adnexal mass with thickened, irregularly-shaped walls

Adnexal mass with irregular solid components

Complex adnexal mass with large cystic component (>10 cm)

Adnexal cyst with multiple internal septations

Multiple, small, irregular peritoneal lesions representing metastases (peritoneal seeding)

Ascites

Peritoneal gelatinous material from pseudomyxoma peritonei suggesting mucin-secreting adenocarcinoma of the ovary

◆ KEY POINTS ◆

1. Ovarian neoplasms are grouped according to the cell type of origin.

2. Primary ovarian neoplasms arise in germ cells, stromal cells, or epithelial cells (75%).

3. Other tumors of the ovaries include lymphoma and metastases from neoplasms of the breasts, uterus and upper gastrointestinal tumors (Krukenberg tumors).

4. Ovarian neoplasms are often silent until they are at an advanced stage, with 65% of patients having metastatic disease at the time of diagnosis.

5. Patients often present with complaints of weight loss, abdominal distension, pelvic discomfort, or pelvic mass.

6. The most common ultrasonographic finding with ovarian carcinoma is a unilateral, complex adnexal mass.

7. Mixed cystic and solid lesions suggest malignancy and are commonly ovarian cystadenocarcinomas.

8. The presence of ascites increases the probability of malignancy.

ENDOMETRIAL CARCINOMA

Anatomy

The uterus normally measures between 6 and 8 cm in length in premenopausal women. In post-menopausal women the uterus may decrease slightly in size to between 4 and 6 cm in length. The endometrial stripe, referred to as the endometrial echo complex (EEC) on ultrasound exams, lines the endometrial canal and should measure no more than 14 mm in thickness if the patient is premenopausal or 5 mm if she is postmenopausal. Patients on tamoxifen therapy may have a slightly increased endometrial stripe, but any patient with an EEC greater than 15 mm should undergo further workup to exclude malignancy.

Etiology

The endometrium normally proliferates during the mid-menstrual cycle. In post-menopausal women the endometrium becomes atrophic and should not continue to proliferate. Abnormal proliferation of the endometrium may occur due to unopposed estrogen or result from adenocarcinoma or sarcoma.

Epidemiology

Endometrial carcinoma is the most common gynecologic malignancy, with 35,000 new cases per year in the United States. Women in their 50s and 60s are most commonly affected. For the less common endometrial sarcoma, there is a wider range for the age of incidence, between 40 and 60. Risk factors for both are related to increased estrogen states and include: early menarche, late menopause, estrogen replacement therapy, obesity, ovulation failure, and nulliparity.

History

Postmenopausal bleeding is the most common presenting symptom. Other symptoms include vague pelvic pain due to increasing uterine size.

Physical Exam

Blood in the cervical os is often noted on gynecologic exam. With sarcoma, prolapsing tissue may be seen. The Pap smear may be helpful if positive but does not exclude the disease if negative. An enlarged uterus or uterine myomas are frequently palpated.

Diagnostic Evaluation

Transvaginal ultrasound is the imaging modality of choice. CT may be helpful in the staging of confirmed cases, but is not as accurate as MRI. Myomata are frequently visualized with CT and MRI and may be indistinguishable from uterine malignancy. The differential diagnosis in women with post-menopausal bleeding should also include bleeding uterine fibroids, endometrial hyperplasia, endometrial polyps, cervical cancer with bleeding, endometriosis, and side effects of estrogen replacement.

Radiologic Findings

A thickened, echogenic (bright on ultrasound) endometrial echo complex that measures more than 15 mm in pre-menopausal women or more than 5 mm in a postmenopausal patient is suggestive of endometrial carcinoma (Figure 7-7). Endometrial hyperplasia or polyps have a similar appearance. An irregular, ill-defined endometrial contour is suspicious for carcinoma. An extension of the echogenic endometrial tissue into or beyond the myometrium is suspicious for malignancy, although adenomyosis (endometriosis of the uterus) may have a similar appearance. CT imaging of endometrial cancer often shows a mass, endometrial enhancement, and fluid within the endometrial canal (Figures 7-8). A dilated canal with fluid may result from uterine tumor obstructing the internal os of the cervix, cervical cancer, an endometrial polyp, or inflammation at the cervical os. Uterine enlargement is a nonspecific finding which may also be seen with a fibroids and adenomyosis.

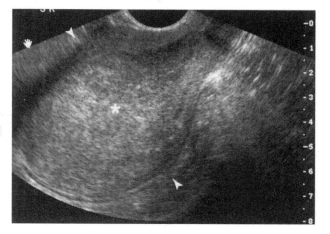

Figure 7-7. Endometrial carcinoma. Thickened, echogenic endometrium (asterisk) on ultrasound of the pelvis. (Used with permission of Cedars-Sinai Medical Center, Los Angeles, California.)

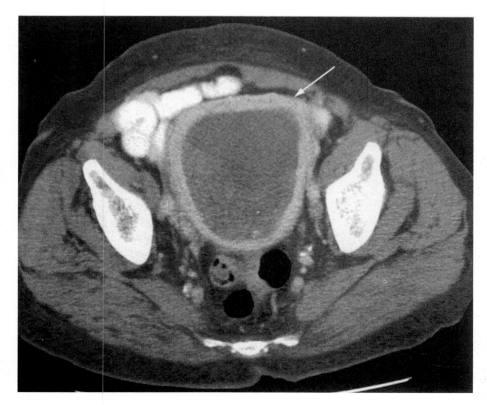

Figure 7-8. Endometrial carcinoma. CT of the pelvis showing dilated endometrial cavity with heterogeneous fluid. (Used with permission of Cedars-Sinai Medical Center, Los Angeles, California.)

◆ KEY POINTS ◆

1. The endometrial stripe, best seen with ultrasound, is the lining of the endometrial canal and should measure no more than 14 mm if the patient is premenopausal or 5 mm if post-menopausal.

2. Post-menopausal bleeding is the most common presenting symptom of endometrial malignancy.

3. Transvaginal ultrasound is the imaging modality of choice.

4. A thickened, irregular, ill-defined endometrial echo complex that measures more than 5 mm (pre-menopausal) or more than 5 mm (post-menopausal) is highly suggestive of endometrial carcinoma.

5. Fluid within the endometrial canal usually is the result of blood. If the canal is dilated, it suggests an obstructing lesion at the internal os, which may be due to endometrial cancer, cervical cancer, endometrial polyp, or inflammation of the cervical os.

8

Musculoskeletal Imaging

TRAUMA

Colles' Fracture

Anatomy

Radiographic description of fractures follows a systematic approach. First, determine the affected bones and anatomic location of each, e.g., epiphysis, metaphysis, or diaphysis. The diaphysis is divided into proximal, middle, and distal portions. Next, describe the pattern of the fracture as simple (two fracture ends, no fragments) or comminuted (more than two fragments). Fracture planes are transverse, oblique, spiral, or longitudinal. Other important features are angulation of the distal fragment, over-riding or distracted fragments, and involvement of the growth plate or joint space.

Colles' fracture, by definition, involves the head of the radius with dorsal angulation of the distal fracture fragment. There is an associated ulnar styloid fracture in approximately 50% of cases.

Etiology

The most common cause is a traumatic fall onto an outstretched hand with the wrist in partial dorsiflexion (Figure 8-1). Force vectors are directed to the distal radius dorsally and proximally.

Epidemiology

The Colles' fracture is the most common fracture of the distal forearm. Osteoporosis increases the risk of occurrence, and classically patients are women over age 70 with some degree of osteoporosis.

History

Patients commonly give a history of a fall while walking. Uneven pavement or misplaced steps frequently cause a person to fall forward and extend the arms in a reflexive action. If a patient cannot recall the cause of the fall, an underlying reason such as ataxia, dehydration, orthostatic hypotension, or syncope should be investigated.

Physical Exam

There is point tenderness over the distal radius and commonly over the ulnar styloid. Soft tissue swelling is

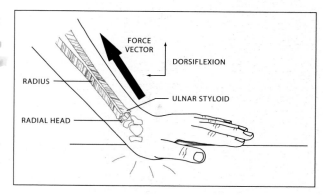

Figure 8-1. Fall onto outstretched hand and mechanism of Colles' fracture. (Illustration by Shawn Girsberger Graphic Design.)

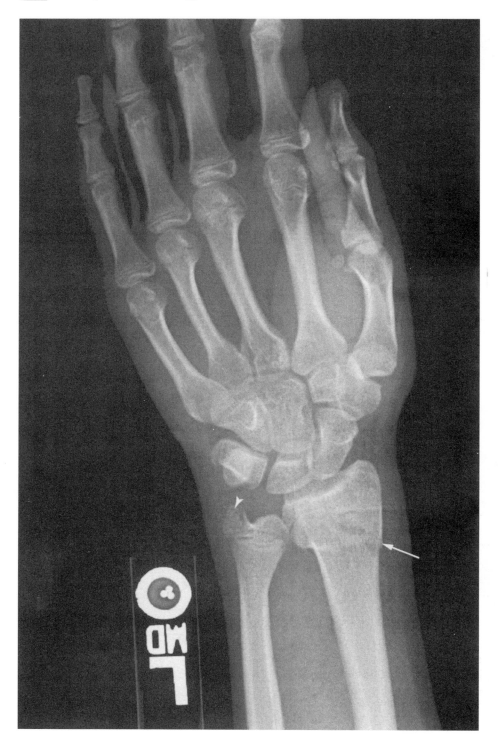

Figures 8-2, 8-3. Colles' fracture AP and lateral views. There is a fracture of the distal radius with mild dorsal angulation of the distal fragment. (Used with permission of Cedars-Sinai Medical Center, Los Angeles, California.)

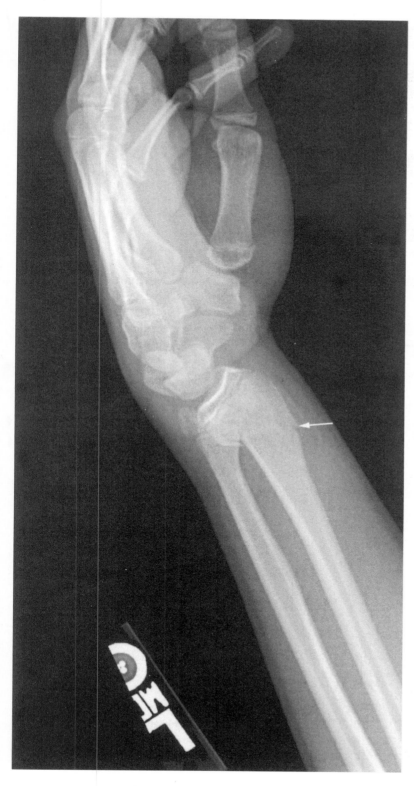

Figure 8-3.

present over the radial aspect of the wrist. The radial pulse should be compared to the contralateral wrist and sensory and motor function of the hand tested. The median and ulnar nerves and the radial artery are rarely affected, but may require surgery if vascular or neurologic compromise is severe.

Diagnostic Evaluation

AP, oblique, and lateral plain radiographs of the distal forearm and wrist are the screening exam of choice for a patient with a suspected Colles' fracture.

Radiologic Findings

Fracture of distal radius with dorsal angulation is the pathognomonic finding for a Colles' fracture (Figures 8-2, 8-3). Typically, a fracture line is seen on the AP view. The lateral view demonstrates the dorsal angulation of the distal radius. Subtle fractures may only be detected as a discontinuity in the normal dense cortical outline. Soft tissue swelling is an important associated finding, as it almost always accompanies a fracture. If there is impaction of the radial head, the radius appears foreshortened. An ulnar styloid fracture is seen in approximately 50% of cases.

A Smith fracture (Figure 8-4) is similar to a Colles' fracture, but there is volar rather than dorsal angulation of the distal radial fragment.

◆ KEY POINTS ◆

1. A Colles' fracture is defined as a fracture of the radial head with dorsal angulation of the distal fragment.
2. Patients give a history of falling onto outstretched hands.

Torus Fracture

Anatomy

A torus or "buckle" fracture may occur in any long bone, but generally is seen in the radius or tibia.

Etiology

Torus fractures generally occur as a result of "buckling" of the cortex due to excessive angulated forces.

Trauma such as jumping from a height greater than six feet or a fall onto outstretched hands may lead to a torus fracture in children aged 5 to 10. Children are susceptible to this type of fracture because the elasticity of their maturing bones causes deformity of the cortex, rather than a fracture along a single plane as in adults.

History

Generally, torus fractures occur after a fall onto an outstretched hand or jumping onto a hard surface from a height. This usually happens during sports or during play such as skateboarding, rollerblading, or bicycling.

Diagnostic Evaluation

AP, lateral, and oblique radiographs of the affected limb are usually sufficient for the diagnosis. Occasionally, radiographs of the contralateral limb are useful for comparison.

Radiologic Findings

The torus or "buckle" fracture is seen as a curved disruption of the cortex and rupture of the periosteum on the convex side, which may extend for a few millimeters up to about 1 cm. The fracture is best seen when it is in profile (Figure 8-5) as opposed to *en face*, and for this reason it is important to obtain three views of the wrist in an attempt to view the fracture at an angle. There is usually mild to moderate overlying soft tissue swelling and tenderness over the suspected area.

◆ KEY POINTS ◆

1. A torus or "buckle" fracture may occur in any long bone, but generally is seen in the radius or tibia.
2. The torus fracture commonly occurs in children ages 5 to 10 after fall onto outstretched hands in the radius or a fall from a height in the tibia.
3. The torus refers to the curved disruption of the cortex and periosteum, without a distinct transverse fracture line.

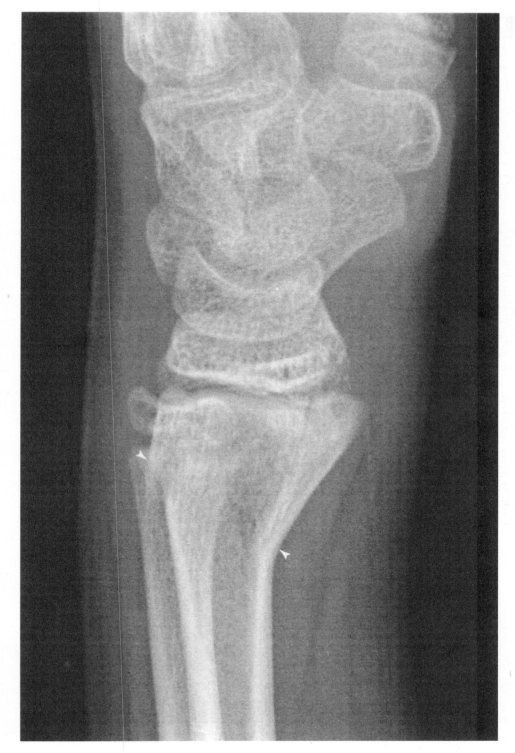

Figure 8-4. Smith fracture. Fracture of the distal radius with volar angulation of the distal fragment.
(Used with permission of Cedars-Sinai Medical Center, Los Angeles, California.)

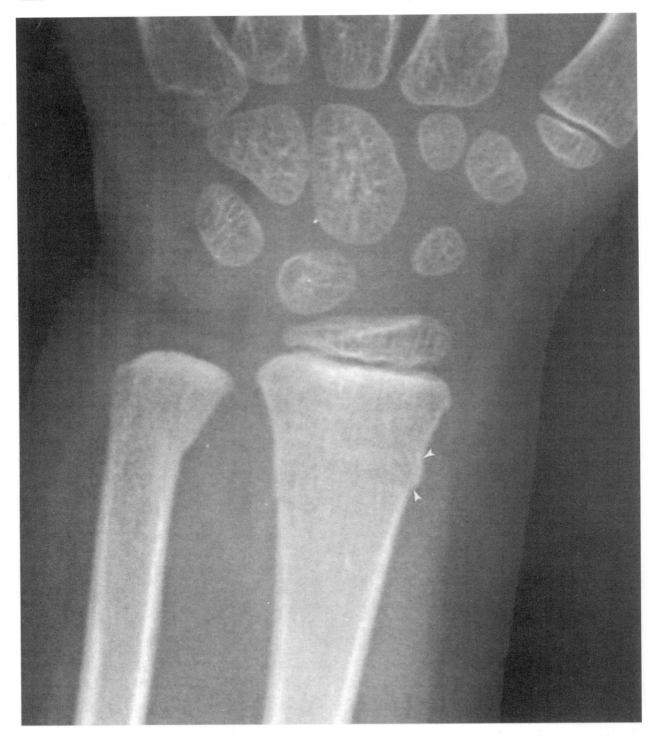

Figure 8-5. Torus fracture of the distal radius in a 10-year-old child who fell while rollerblading. Notice the buckle in the radial metaphysis on the AP view (arrowheads). (Used with permission of Cedars-Sinai Medical Center, Los Angeles, California.)

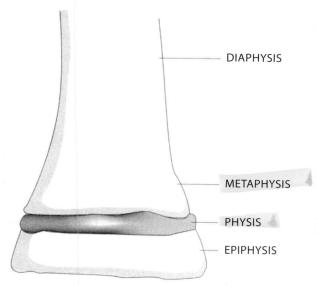

Figure 8-6. Diagram of the anatomy of bone growth plate. (Illustration by Shawn Girsberger Graphic Design.)

Salter-Harris Fracture

Anatomy

The long bones are divided into three sections related to the physis, or growth plate (Figure 8-6). The epiphysis is distal to the physis in the direction of growth; the metaphysis is immediately adjacent to the physis on the opposite side of the epiphysis, and the diaphysis is the long shaft beyond the metaphysis. In growing children with open epiphysial plates, approximately 35% of all skeletal injuries involve the growth plate in some way. The most common sites are the wrist (50%), ankle (30%) and knee. Damaging the physis may cause growth deformities, such as limb length discrepancies and angulations, to occur.

Etiology

Any trauma with sufficient force may cause a fracture or disruption of the growth plate. The injuries are analogous to ligamentous injuries in adults.

Epidemiology

Growth plate injuries account for approximately 35% of all skeletal injuries in children between the ages of 10 and 15. Younger children generally will have greenstick (Figure 8-7) or torus (Figure 8-5) fractures.

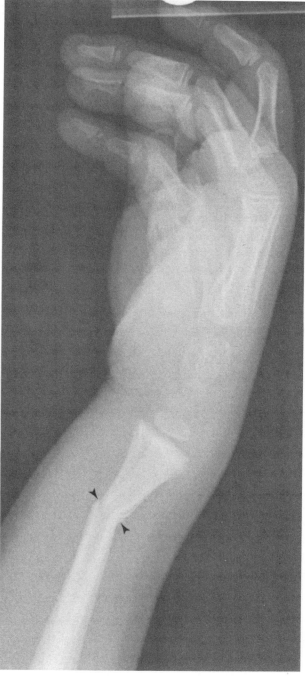

Figure 8-7. Greenstick fracture of the distal radius and ulna. Only the volar cortices have displaced fractures. The dorsal cortices demonstrate a bending type of fracture. (Used with permission of Cedars-Sinai Medical Center, Los Angeles, California.)

History

Patients present following trauma and, in the 10- to 15-year-old age group, this is usually the result of a sports-related injury or a fall. The chief complaint is pain in the affected limb and point tenderness over the fracture.

Physical Exam

Soft tissue swelling overlying the fracture or diffusely over the affected joint is seen on gross examination. A full neurovascular exam should be performed, as Salter-Harris fractures may affect adjacent nerves or vessels.

Diagnostic Evaluation

AP, lateral, and oblique radiographs of the affected joint are standard for screening of suspected fractures. CT scan of the affected limb may be obtained if intra-articular involvement is suspected but not definite on the plain films. MRI is rarely indicated but may show marrow edema and prove non-displaced fractures not evident on screening radiographs.

Radiologic Findings

Salter-Harris fractures are classified into five types (Figure 8-8). The mnemonic of SALTR describes each type as: slipped, above, lower, through, and ruined.

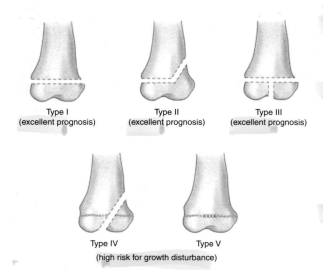

Type I
(excellent prognosis)

Type II
(excellent prognosis)

Type III
(excellent prognosis)

Type IV   Type V
(high risk for growth disturbance)

Figure 8-8. Epiphysial fractures: Salter-Harris classification. (Illustration by Electronic Illustrators Group.)

Type I (5%): "Slipped" or displaced physis

Type II (75%): Fracture above the physis, involving the metaphysis (Figures 8-9, 8-10)

Type III (10%): Fracture below the physis, involving only the epiphysis

Type IV (10%): Fracture through the metaphysis, physis, and epiphysis (Figure 8-11)

Type V (rare <1%): Crush injury to the physis

◆ KEY POINTS ◆

1. Salter-Harris fractures are classified into five types. The mnemonic of SALTR describes each type as: slipped, above, lower, through, and ruined.

2. These fractures affect children between the ages of 10 and 15.

3. AP, lateral, and oblique radiographs of the affected joint are standard for screening of suspected fractures.

Hip Fracture

Anatomy

Femoral fractures usually occur at one of three areas: subcapital, intertrochanteric or subtrochanteric (Figure 8-12). Subtrochanteric fractures are usually associated with more severe trauma and are more common in men. The circumflex artery of the femur, which supplies the femoral head, may be affected, especially with subcapital fractures. Avascular necrosis of the femoral head is a complication of 10 to 30% of subcapital fractures.

Etiology

The underlying etiology is commonly either osteoporosis or chronic systemic steroid use. Acute fractures are usually due to trauma, but osteoporotic fractures without associated major trauma have been reported. Pathologic fractures may occur as a result of metastatic lesions or primary bone lesions.

Epidemiology

The incidence of hip fracture is approximately 200,000 cases per year in the United States. Patients are predominantly postmenopausal women, but men with osteoporosis and any patient taking steroids

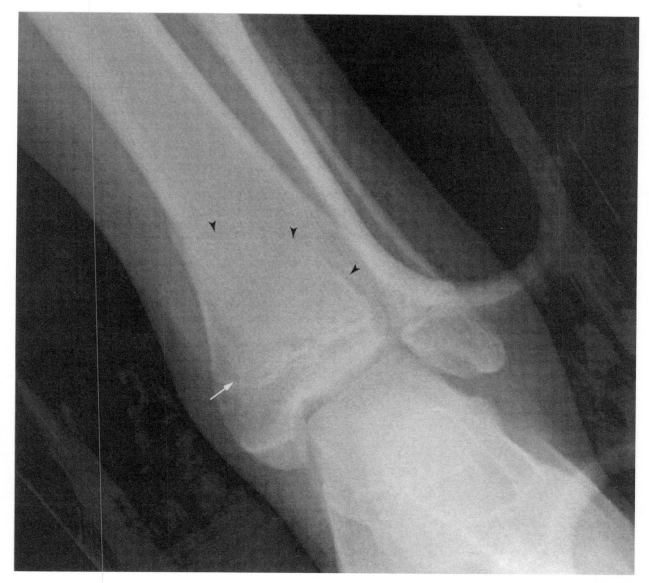

Figures 8-9, 8-10. AP and lateral views of Salter-Harris II fracture of the left ankle in a 12-year-old boy. The fracture line involves the distal tibial metaphysis. (Used with permission of Cedars-Sinai Medical Center, Los Angeles, California.)

chronically for other conditions are at increased risk. Inadequate calcium and vitamin D intake, lack of exercise, and alcohol use are predisposing factors.

History

Pain is noted in the groin area of the affected side. Severe pain is suggestive of a displaced fracture. Patients may complain of pain at rest, but most when attempting to weight-bear.

Physical Exam

External rotation and shortening of the affected leg is often noted on gross examination. Pain is elicited on motion of the hip and there may be referred pain to the knee.

Diagnostic Evaluation

Beyond the history and physical exam, an AP radiograph of the pelvis and AP and "frog-leg" (abduction and external rotation) lateral views of the affected hip should

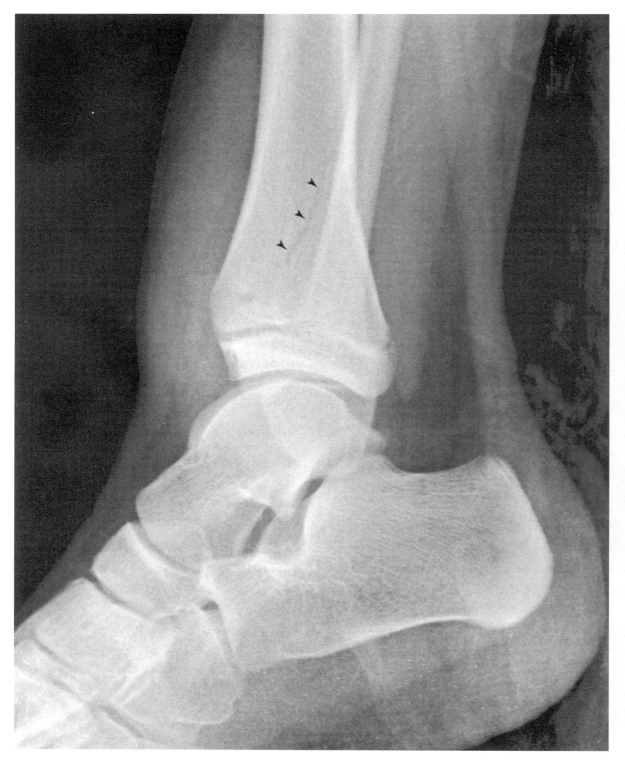

Figure 8-10.

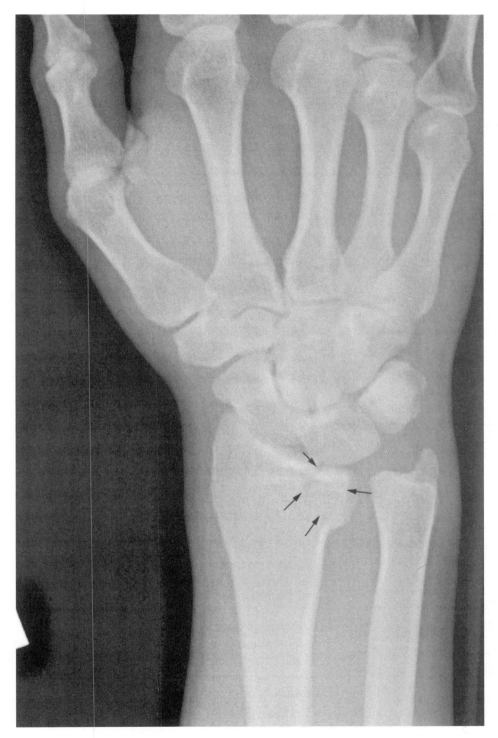

Figure 8-11. Salter-Harris type IV fracture that extends through the physis in the right radius of a 9-year-old boy. (Used with permission of Cedars-Sinai Medical Center, Los Angeles, California.)

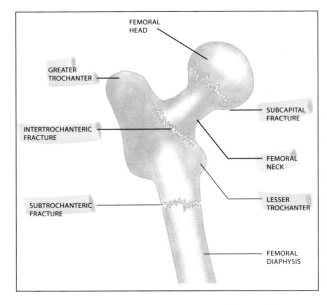

Figure 8-12. Diagram of common points of femoral fracture. (Illustration by Shawn Girsberger Graphic Design.)

◆ KEY POINTS ◆

1. Fractures of the hip usually occur at one of three places: subcapital, intertrochanteric, and subtrochanteric.

2. Underlying etiology is most commonly osteoporosis due to age or chronic steroid use. Pathologic fractures may occur as a result of metastatic lesions or primary bone lesions.

3. AP radiograph of the pelvis and AP and "frogleg" lateral views of the affected hip should be obtained.

be obtained. AP and lateral films of the femur and knee may be ordered to exclude other fractures and to exclude other causes of referred pain into the knee. Another important test is the post-reduction film, which is used to exclude fracture fragments not seen on initial films and to confirm adequate fracture reduction to avoid non-union.

Radiologic Findings

Fractures often are seen as a disruption of the cortex, as a lucent fracture line (Figure 8-13), or as an offset of the normal anatomic alignment of the femur, if the fracture is displaced. With subcapital fractures, there is often angulation of the femoral head compared to the contralateral side. Nondisplaced fractures may not have any plain film radiographic evidence. For this reason, they are often referred to as occult fractures. If the clinical picture is suspicious, but plain films are negative, MRI or radionuclide bone scan is useful. Findings on MRI include linear decreased signal intensity on T1-weighted images, signifying a fracture line. Nuclear scintigraphy is useful after the healing phase begins and radionuclide taken up by osteoblasts demonstrates increased activity, i.e., a "hot-spot" on Technetium bone scan.

Rheumatoid Arthritis

Epidemiology

Rheumatoid arthritis is the most common of the inflammatory arthritides. The underlying pathology is the formation of pannus, the overproduction of synovial tissue, which fills joint spaces and erodes articular cartilage and bone. The age distribution is from 25 to 55, with a peak in the 20 to 30 range. The ratio of women to men is approximately 3:1. There is also an association with HLA-DW4.

Diagnosis

Patients have chief complaint of joint pain and stiffness, worse in the morning, lasting at least one hour. The detection of rheumatoid factor (RF) in the serum is helpful in making the diagnosis, though not essential, as 20% of patients may have "sero-negative" arthritis. These include Reiter's syndrome, psoriatic arthritis, and ankylosing spondylitis. Extra-articular manifestations that may aid in the diagnosis include rheumatoid nodules (20 to 25%), vasculitis, scleritis, pericarditis, pleural effusions, and interstitial lung fibrosis.

Radiologic Findings

Posterior-anterior plain films of the hands and wrists remain the gold standard in both the diagnosis and the follow-up of rheumatoid arthritis. Common radiographic findings include:

• Classic joint deformities such as swan-neck deformity of the PIP and DIP joints of the hands (Figure 8-14), Boutonnière deformity of the phalanges, and ulnar deviation of the wrist

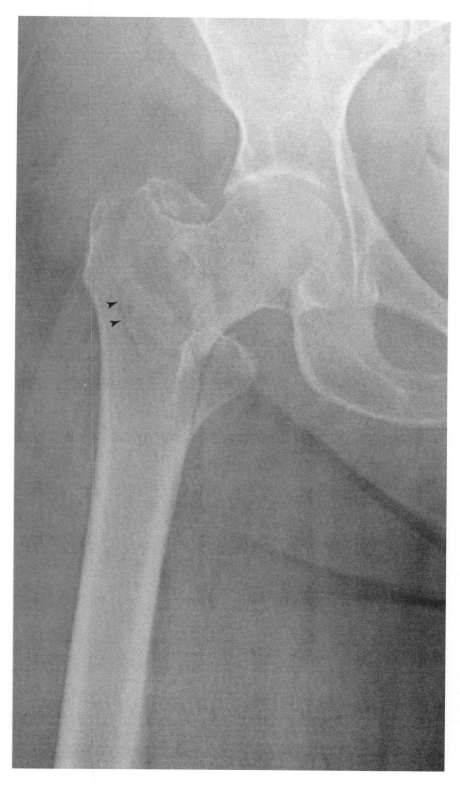

Figure 8-13. Hip fracture. Intertrochanteric fracture in the right hip of an 83-year-old woman who fell after getting out of bed. (Used with permission of Cedars-Sinai Medical Center, Los Angeles, California.)

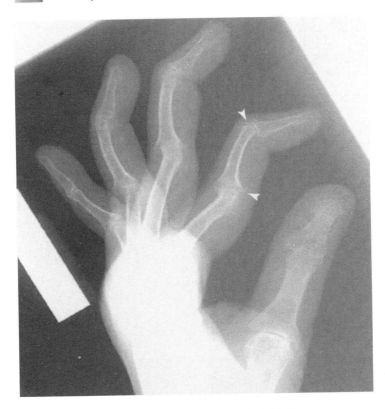

Figure 8-14. Rheumatoid arthritis. Classic swan-neck deformity of the hands. Hyperextension of PIP joint and hyperflexion of DIP joint. (Used with permission of Cedars-Sinai Medical Center, Los Angeles, California.)

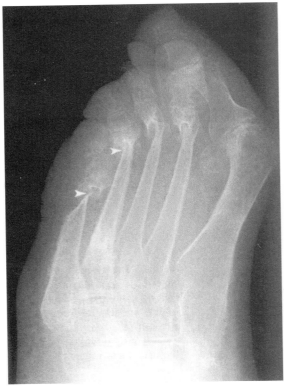

Figure 8-15. Periarticular erosions in the metatarsal-phalangeal joints. (Used with permission of Cedars-Sinai Medical Center, Los Angeles, California.)

- Periarticular osteopenia (early finding) and erosions (late finding) (Figure 8-15)
- Osseous erosions located away from the weight-bearing area of the affected joint
- Uniform joint space narrowing caused by loss of cartilage from invading pannus
- Polyarticular, symmetric joint involvement (MCP, MTP, carpal, tarsal, acromioclavicular, hip, atlantoaxial joint)
- Soft tissue swelling

◆ **KEY POINTS** ◆

1. Radiologic diagnosis is made with PA plain films of the hands and wrists.
2. Findings include: soft tissue swelling, periarticular osteopenia, joint space narrowing, and classic deformities of the fingers and wrists.
3. Rheumatoid arthritis is classically bilateral and symmetric.
4. Extra-articular manifestations may aid in the diagnosis.

9

Pediatric Imaging

FOREIGN BODY ASPIRATION

Anatomy

A foreign body that is aspirated into the airway is usually a small object (most commonly a small piece of food, a peanut, a coin, or a small toy) that is inhaled rather than swallowed. Normally, the epiglottis prevents aspiration by covering the laryngeal vestibule and diverting food into the esophagus. Sites of obstruction are almost exclusively the lower lobe bronchi, most commonly the right mainstem bronchus.

Etiology

In the normal course of development, children ages 1 to 3 tend to investigate objects by placing them in their mouths. Developmentally, this is a vulnerable time as they may aspirate the object into the airway when inhaling normally.

Pathogenesis

Acute obstruction of the airway prevents oxygenation of the affected lung. Without airflow, the obstructed portion of lung will collapse. Chronic obstruction leads to pneumonia and bronchiectasis.

Epidemiology

Children less than age 3 are most susceptible to foreign body aspiration, because they tend to play with small objects and frequently place them in their mouth. Toys should be inspected for small removable parts. Coins, keys, stones, and foods such as nuts and peas should be avoided because of their small size and frequent association with airway obstruction.

History

Children often present with the sudden onset of wheezing, choking, or respiratory distress while playing or eating. With partial obstruction, they are able to cough and often have acute wheezing. In complete obstruction, they may have shortness of breath, tachypnea, and hypoxemia. If the obstruction is prolonged, loss of consciousness may result from the oxygen deprivation.

Physical Exam

On auscultation, there is often absent or decreased breath sounds on the side of the obstruction. Use of accessory muscles of respiration is noted as the child struggles to aerate the lungs. Grunting and wheezing are common. The oropharynx should be inspected in an attempt to visualize the obstructing object that could potentially be removed. Oxygen saturation on pulse oximetry is reduced.

Diagnostic Evaluation

When a foreign body airway obstruction is suspected, the primary screening study is the frontal chest x-ray with right and left decubitus views. Fluoroscopic examination of the lungs may be performed if the radiographs

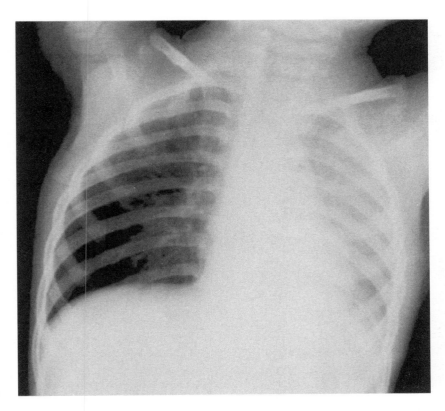

Figure 9-1. Foreign body aspiration. Hyperlucency of the right lung on expiration. The left lung has compressive changes normal for an expiratory film. This patient had a peanut in the right mainstem bronchus. (Used with permission of Cedars-Sinai Medical Center, Los Angeles, California.)

are equivocal. CT of the chest is not typically performed, but may be helpful in demonstrating the object if coronal reformations are included. Direct visualization with endoscopy may be needed because up to 30% of cases with negative radiologic findings turn out to be positive.

Radiologic Findings

With bronchial obstruction, the most common finding is hyperlucency of the lung on the affected side due to air trapping (Figure 9-1). The obstructing object acts as a ball-valve, allowing air to enter the lung but not to escape. On decubitus views, the lung on the side that the patient is laying is more collapsed than the non-dependent lung. When both decubitus views are obtained, the lung with the obstruction remains hyperinflated on both views (Figures 9-2, 9-3). Less commonly in bronchial obstruction there may be atelectasis of all or part of the lung distal to the obstruction.

In upper airway obstruction of the larynx or trachea, the chest x-ray may appear normal or with bilateral hyperinflation of the lungs.

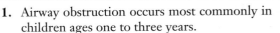

◆ KEY POINTS ◆

1. Airway obstruction occurs most commonly in children ages one to three years.

2. Presenting symptoms are sudden onset of choking, gagging, or coughing.

3. The most common radiologic finding is hyperlucency and hyperinflation of the lung on the affected side due to air trapping.

RESPIRATORY DISTRESS SYNDROME

Anatomy

Respiratory distress syndrome (RDS) is the most common cause of respiratory distress in neonates. In the normal lung, the alveoli are coated with surfactant that prevents the airspaces from collapsing during expiration. In respiratory distress syndrome the alveoli are poorly formed and collapsed, not allowing the proper exchange of oxygen with the bloodstream.

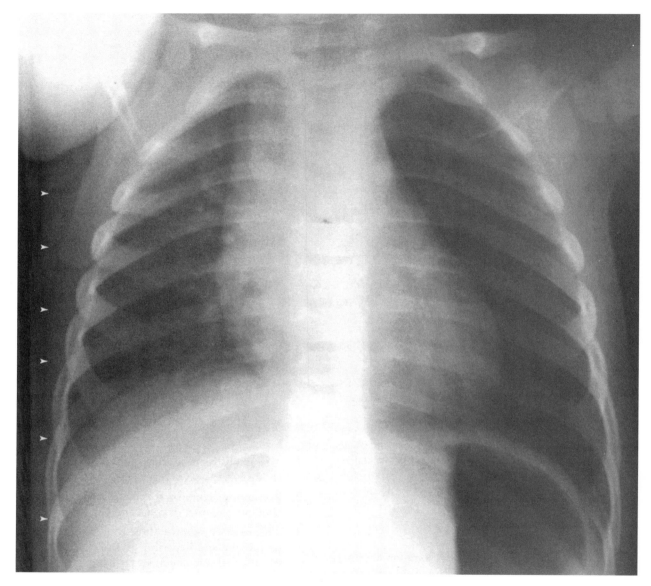

Figures 9-2, 9-3. Foreign body aspiration. Right lateral decubitus view of the chest shows that the right lung compresses normally when it is dependent (Figure 9-2). Compare to left lateral decubitus view (Figure 9-3), where the left lung remains hyperinflated although it is the dependent lung (arrowheads point to dependent side). This indicates a left mainstem bronchus foreign body. The patient inhaled a small plastic building block. (Used with permission of Cedars-Sinai Medical Center, Los Angeles, California.)

Etiology

RDS, also known as hyaline membrane disease, is caused by a deficiency in alveolar surfactant. Type II pneumocytes begin producing surfactant at 24 weeks gestational age and peak production occurs at 36 weeks. Without surfactant, surface tension within alveoli increases and atelectasis occurs during expiration. Increasing inspiratory pressures are required to expand the alveoli.

Pathogenesis

The surfactant deficiency results in collapsed alveoli, decreased oxygenation, and pulmonary vasoconstriction.

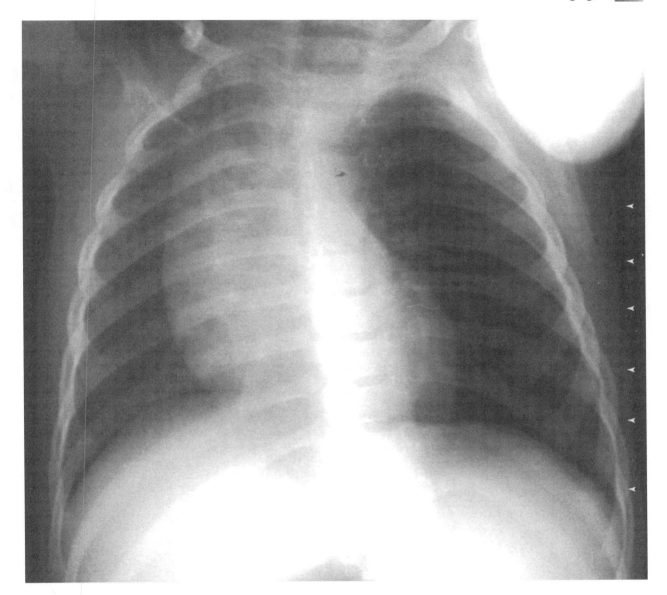

Figure 9-3.

This in turn leads to capillary damage and leak of plasma into the alveoli, which combines with fibrin and necrotic pneumocytes to form the proteinaceous material called "hyaline membranes" in the airspaces. The hyaline membranes prevent oxygen from diffusing across the alveolar membrane, leading to further hypoxemia and respiratory distress.

Epidemiology

The risk of RDS correlates with prematurity of the neonate. Fifty percent of all newborns born at 28 weeks will have RDS. The incidence decreases as the gestational age increases. For term infants, the incidence is less than five percent. For this reason, RDS should be high on the differential diagnosis for premature neonates and low for full-term infants.

History

The onset of increasing dyspnea and hypoxia one to two hours after birth is the most common presentation. Usually, the infant is intubated due to increasing oxygen requirement.

Physical Exam

Tachypnea, grunting, nasal flaring, chest retractions, and cyanosis are noted within the first two hours after birth. Breath sounds are decreased bilaterally due to poor air entry.

Diagnostic Evaluation

If the history and physical findings are consistent with RDS, arterial blood gas sampling should be performed to determine the severity of hypoxemia. A stat chest radiograph is obtained to exclude pneumonia, pneumothorax, or other causes of respiratory distress in the newborn. Intubation and mechanical ventilation are often necessary. If RDS is indeed the cause, the infant will eventually require mechanical ventilation.

Radiologic Findings

RDS is suspected in any premature infant with any opacification in the lungs. Diagnosis cannot be based on a single chest x-ray, especially if the infant is not intubated. Diffuse "ground-glass" or reticulogranular opacifications are most common (Figure 9-4). Low lung volumes are often present initially, especially prior to

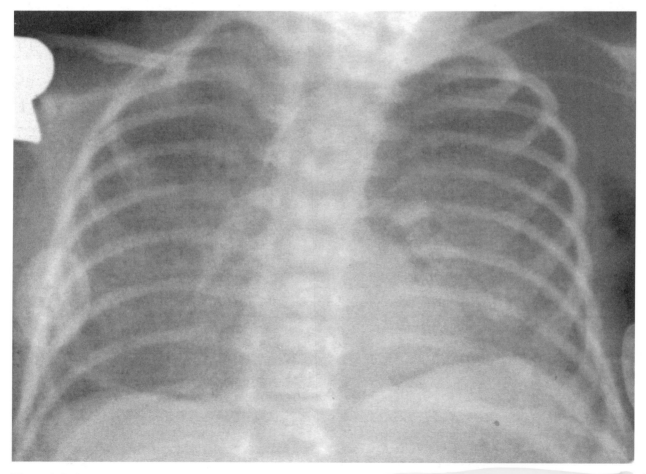

Figure 9-4. Respiratory distress syndrome. This AP chest radiograph reveals low lung volumes and diffuse ground-glass opacification in a premature baby born at 30 weeks gestation. (Used with permission of Cedars-Sinai Medical Center, Los Angeles, California.)

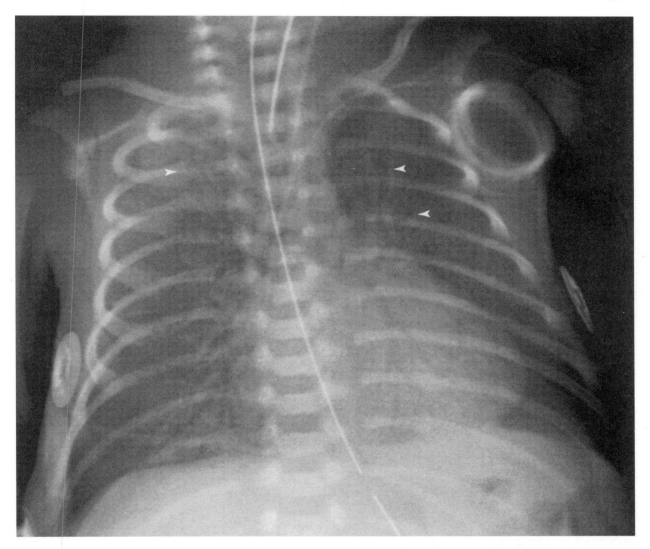

Figure 9-5. Respiratory distress syndrome. This patient is intubated and there are diffuse ground-glass opacifications consistent with respiratory distress syndrome. Subtle tortuous lucencies represent pulmonary interstitial emphysema. (Used with permission of Cedars-Sinai Medical Center, Los Angeles, California.)

intubation. Follow-up films often reveal progression to air-trapping with pulmonary interstitial emphysema (Figure 9-5), an accumulation of gas in the peribronchial spaces, and increasing diffuse opacities approaching whiteout of the lungs. The differential diagnosis includes pneumonia, pulmonary edema, and transient tachypnea of the newborn (Figures 9-6a, b) a condition in which there is residual pulmonary fluid which gradually clears after two to three days. Complications of RDS include pneumothorax (Figures 9-7a, b) and

pneumomediastinum (Figure 9-7c) due to the decreased compliance of the alveoli and the high pulmonary pressures needed to oxygenate the patients.

DUODENAL STENOSIS

Anatomy

The C-loop of the duodenum normally lies posterior and to the right of the pylorus of the stomach. It traverses

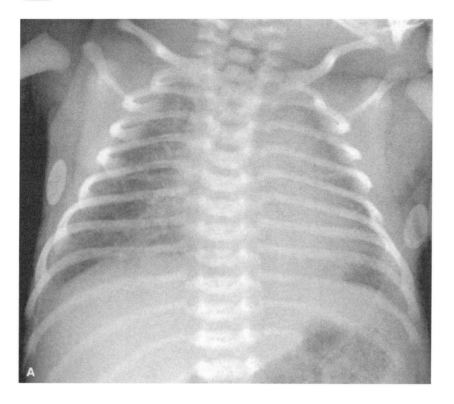

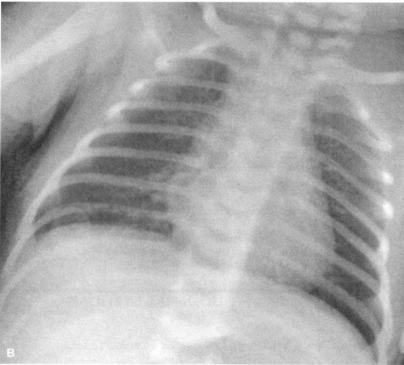

Figure 9-6a, b. Transient tachypnea of the newborn. The chest radiograph of a full-term infant in 9-6a reveals diffuse parenchymal opacification that cleared on the follow-up film taken three days later (9-6b). (Used with permission of Cedars-Sinai Medical Center, Los Angeles, California.)

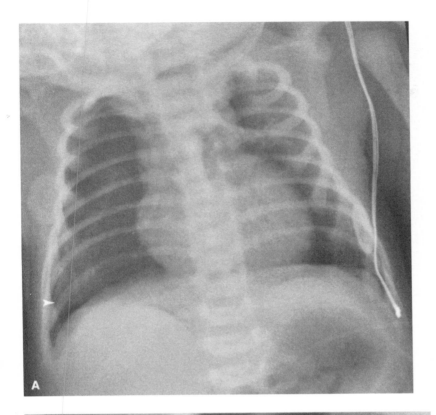

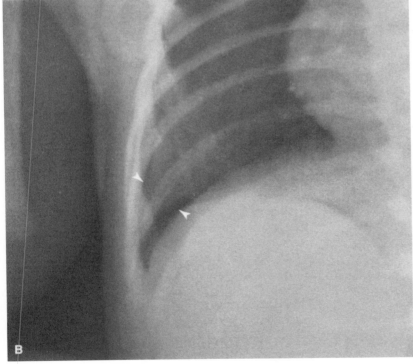

Figure 9-7a, b. Pneumothorax. An area of lucency is seen in the right lower thorax near the right costophrenic angle (9-7b magnification view). This was a complication of long-standing RDS. (Used with permission of Cedars-Sinai Medical Center, Los Angeles, California.)

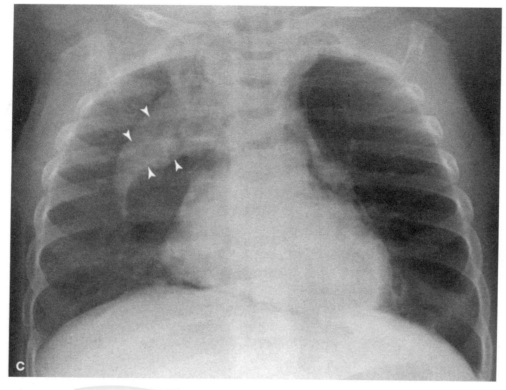

Figure 9-7c. Pneumomediastinum. This patient had been intubated for RDS and developed pneumomediastinum from barotrauma. Note the elevation of the right portion of the thymus, a finding commonly called the "sail sign." (Used with permission of Cedars-Sinai Medical Center, Los Angeles, California.)

◆ **KEY POINTS** ◆

1. Respiratory distress syndrome, also known as hyaline membrane disease, is caused by a deficiency in alveolar surfactant.
2. The risk of RDS increases with increasing prematurity of the neonate.
3. Diffuse ground-glass or reticulonodular opacifications are most common.

---

back to the left and the Ligament of Treitz is normally left of the midline.

Etiology

Duodenal stenosis is caused by failure of recanalization of the duodenum during embryologic development, which normally occurs at 10 weeks gestation.

Epidemiology

The incidence is approximately 1:3500 live births. There is a 30% association of duodenal atresia and Down syndrome. Duodenal stenosis and atresia commonly present within 24 hours of birth.

History

Classically, the history is a newborn with bilious vomiting and inability to tolerate feeding due to the obstruction. The vomiting is non-projectile compared to pyloric stenosis, which presents with non-bilious projectile vomiting after each feeding.

Physical Exam

Abdominal distension is often noted, which represents the distended stomach. Often the exam may be normal. Imperforate anus is associated with a small percentage of cases.

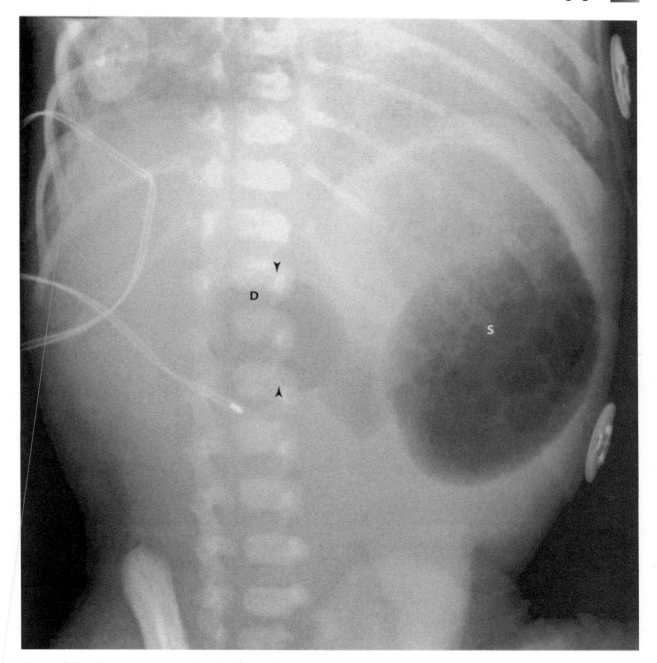

Figure 9-8a. Duodenal stenosis. AP radiograph of the abdomen of a child who presented with bilious vomiting. The image reveals a classic "double-bubble" sign, which represents the stomach (S) and the duodenal bulb (D), filled with gas and secretions. (Used with permission of Cedars-Sinai Medical Center, Los Angeles, California.)

Diagnostic Evaluation

The differential diagnosis of a "double-bubble" sign on an abdominal radiograph includes duodenal atresia, duodenal stenosis, annular pancreas, and midgut volvulus.

Radiologic Findings

The classic finding is the "double-bubble" sign, which represents the dilated stomach and duodenal bulb (Figures 9-8a, b). Air cannot pass beyond the duodenum

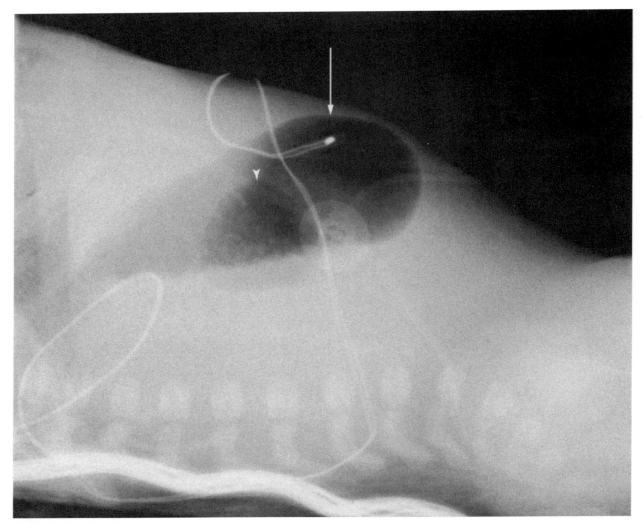

Figure 9-8b. Duodenal stenosis. Cross-table lateral view reveals gas in the stomach (arrow) that is anterior to the duodenal bulb (arrowhead), also filled with gas. Notice that there is a paucity of gas in the rest of the abdomen. (Used with permission of Cedars-Sinai Medical Center, Los Angeles, California.)

so there is a paucity of bowel gas throughout the abdomen.

MECONIUM ASPIRATION

Etiology

Meconium is the sterile intestinal material of the newborn. It contains mucosal epithelial cells, bile, and mucous. Normally, it is passed from the rectum within 12 hours of delivery. Meconium aspiration occurs when the meconium is passed in utero and mixes with the amniotic fluid. Risk factors include post-maturity (>42 weeks gestational age), fetal distress from prolonged labor, premature rupture of membranes, and congenital infection.

Pathogenesis

It is believed that fetal hypoxia from any of the causes listed above triggers a vagal nerve-mediated expulsion of meconium from the GI tract into the amniotic fluid. The aspirated meconium acts as a chemical irritant in the lungs and causes an inflammatory response that varies from mild to severe depending on the amount of aspiration.

◆ KEY POINTS ◆

1. Duodenal atresia is caused by failure of re-canalization of the duodenum during embryologic development.

2. There is a 30% association of duodenal atresia and Down syndrome.

3. The history is a newborn with bilious non-projectile vomiting.

4. The classic radiologic finding is the "double-bubble" sign.

Epidemiology

Passing of meconium into the amniotic fluid occurs in approximately 10% of all live births. Clinically significant meconium aspiration occurs in 10% of these, or approximately 1% of all live births.

History and Physical

Green-colored meconium is noted at birth especially during suctioning of the neonate's airway. Sometimes the aspiration is undetected at birth but suspected as the patient presents with tachypnea and hypoxia. Diffuse, coarse rales are heard on auscultation. The newborn may have

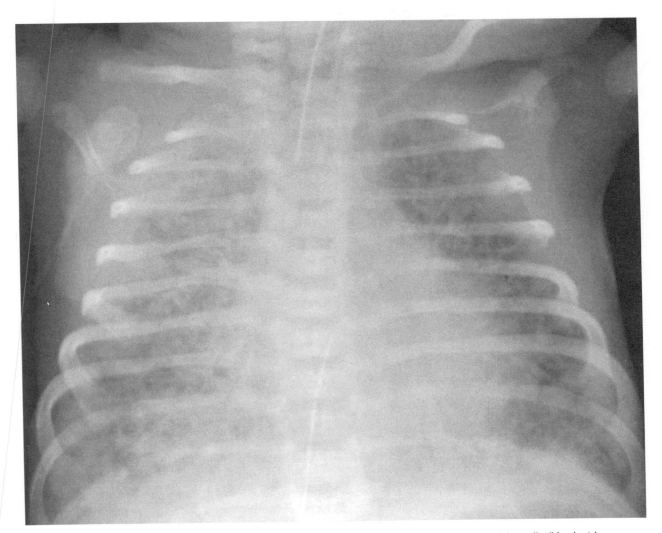

Figure 9-9. Meconium aspiration. AP chest radiograph reveals coarse opacifications of the lungs bilaterally. (Used with permission of Cedars-Sinai Medical Center, Los Angeles, California).

an oxygen requirement that increases as the chemical pneumonitis causes an increased inflammatory reaction.

Diagnostic Evaluation

The chest radiograph is the diagnostic imaging study of choice. Fever should be monitored, blood cultures drawn to exclude infection, and blood gas taken to determine the extent of hypoxemia. Serial daily chest x-rays are obtained until there are signs of resolution. Radiographs commonly seem to worsen the first few days, but begin to clear by five days in most cases.

Radiologic Findings

The most common finding is diffuse patchy opacification of the lungs. The pattern is often described as "coarse" due to the filling of the airspaces with meconium and the surrounding inflammatory reaction (Figure 9-9). The lungs are often hyperinflated and air bronchograms are commonly seen. Pneumothoraces develop as the meconium causes ball-valve obstruction of airways.

◆ KEY POINTS ◆

1. Meconium aspiration occurs when the meconium is passed in utero and mixes with the amniotic fluid.

2. Meconium acts as a chemical irritant in the lungs and causes an inflammatory response.

3. The chest radiograph is the first imaging study that should be performed.

4. The most common finding is diffuse coarse opacification of the lungs.

Questions

1. A 56-year-old man presents to your office with a two-month history of cough, malaise, and weight loss. He has smoked one pack per day for the past 30 years. He denies any fever, chills, or night sweats. What is the next most appropriate diagnostic step?

   A. Chest CT scan

   B. Sputum cultures

   C. PA and lateral chest radiographs

   D. Bronchoscopy

   E. Chest MRI

2. A 20-year-old woman presents to the emergency department following a motor vehicle accident. She was an unrestrained passenger in a head-on collision, and has multiple facial lacerations and contusions. She had been complaining of right hip pain, but now is somewhat somnolent with a Glasgow coma score of 8. What is the next most appropriate diagnostic test?

   A. Contrast-enhanced head CT

   B. Non-contrast head CT

   C. Right hip radiographs

   D. AP pelvis

   E. Cervical spine radiograph series

3. A 42-year-old man presents to your office with complaints of recurrent sinus infections. You treated him one month ago with Amoxicillin/ Clavulanate for acute sinusitis. He returns stating that although the medication did help, the infection never completely resolved. He affirms that he took the entire course of antibiotics. On physical exam, you notice an effusion behind the right tympanic membrane. What is the most appropriate next step?

   A. Culture the nasopharynx

   B. Prescribe a second course of Amoxicillin

   C. Prescribe a course of Azithromycin

   D. Order a contrast-enhanced CT of the neck

   E. Order skull radiographs with Waters and Townes views

4. A 74-year-old man presents to the emergency department with slurred speech and left-sided weakness that began one hour ago. A non-contrast CT scan of the head reveals an area of hypoattenuation in the right frontal lobe. What is the most likely diagnosis?

   A. Hypertensive crisis

   B. Meningitis

   C. Carotid artery dissection

D. Stroke

E. Astrocytoma

5. An 8-year-old boy presents to the emergency department with nausea, vomiting, and abdominal pain. An abdominal ultrasound is performed (Figure Q-5): What is the diagnosis?

A. Crohn's disease

B. Appendicitis

C. Ulcerative colitis

D. Small bowel obstruction

E. Renal colic

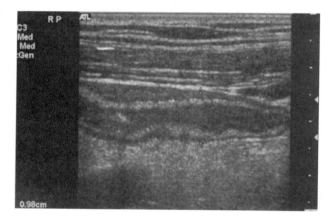

Question 5. (Used with permission of Cedars-Sinai Medical Center, Los Angeles, California.)

6. A 26-year-old woman presents to the emergency department with left lower quadrant pain and tenderness on examination. Beta-HCG is positive. What is the next most appropriate step in managing this patient?

A. Inform the patient that she is pregnant, reassure her that the pain is related to the pregnancy, and send her home with arrangements to follow-up with her primary care physician

B. Obtain a pelvic ultrasound

C. Perform a speculum exam with a cervical culture

D. Order an abdominal/pelvic CT scan

E. Consult obstetrics

7. Which of the following ultrasonographic signs is associated with acute cholecystitis?

A. Fluid around the gallbladder

B. Thickened gallbladder wall

C. Gallbladder distension

D. All of the above

E. None of the above

8. A 60-year-old man with a history of alcoholism comes to your office complaining of intermittent chest pain. A CT scan of the abdomen is shown below (Figure Q-8). What is the most likely diagnosis?

A. Gastric carcinoma

B. Chronic pancreatitis

C. Renal cell carcinoma

D. Aortic aneurysm

E. None of the above.

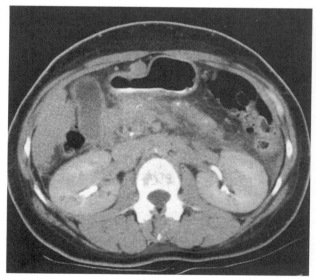

Question 8. (Used with permission of Cedars-Sinai Medical Center, Los Angeles, California.)

9. A 3-year-old boy presents to the emergency department with cough and difficulty breathing. The mother reports that he has had a fever to 100° F and a barking cough since the night before. A chest radiograph is ordered. Which radiologic sign is most useful in making the diagnosis?

   A. Foreign body in the airway

   B. The steeple sign

   C. Deviated trachea

   D. Unilateral lucent hemithorax

   E. Deep sulcus sign

10. In which age group is the following injury (Figure Q-10) most likely to occur?

    A. 2 months

    B. 2 years

    C. 8 years

    D. 20 years

    E. 70 years

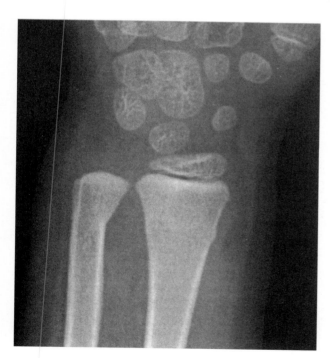

Question 10. (Used with permission of Cedars-Sinai Medical Center, Los Angeles, California.)

11. You are called by a nurse in the hospital to evaluate a 65-year-old woman who is three days status-post hip replacement. She was starting her physical therapy exercises and became short of breath. She is complaining of left-sided chest pain. What is the most sensitive test to establish the diagnosis?

    A. CT scan of the chest with contrast

    B. V/Q scan

    C. Lower extremity Doppler examination

    D. Pulmonary angiogram

    E. EKG

12. A 35-year-old man presents to the emergency department following a stab wound to the right side of the chest. A chest x-ray reveals blunting of the right costophrenic angle. What is the most likely diagnosis?

    A. Pneumothorax

    B. Pneumonia

    C. Hemopericardium

    D. Hemothorax

    E. Pulmonary contusion

13. A 46-year-old woman presents with six hours of intermittent right flank pain radiating to the groin. Urinalysis shows microscopic hematuria. She has a history of Crohn's disease, which has been controlled by steroids in the past. Which of the following is the best test to establish the diagnosis?

    A. Barium enema

    B. Upper gastrointestinal series with small bowel follow-through

    C. Non-contrast CT scan of the abdomen and pelvis

    D. Intravenous pyelogram

    E. Ultrasound of the abdomen

14. A 44-year-old woman comes to your office complaining of increasing menstrual bleeding. On physical examination, you determine that the uterus is enlarged, with irregular contours. You suspect that the bleeding is due to uterine leiomyomas. Which is the most appropriate next step in your management?

    A. CT scan of the pelvis

    B. Ultrasound of the pelvis

C. Abdominal plain radiographs

D. MRI of the pelvis

E. Hysterosalpingogram

15. Which of the following radiologic findings are associated with childhood asthma?

A. Interstitial fibrosis

B. Lobar pneumonia

C. Widened mediastinum

D. Hyperinflated lungs

E. Pneumothorax

16. A 1-day-old girl presents from the nursery with frequent vomiting and abdominal bloating. An abdominal radiograph is obtained (Figure Q-16). What is the diagnosis?

A. Pyloric stenosis

B. Duodenal atresia

C. Necrotizing enterocolitis

D. Hirschsprung's disease

E. Tracheoesophageal fistula

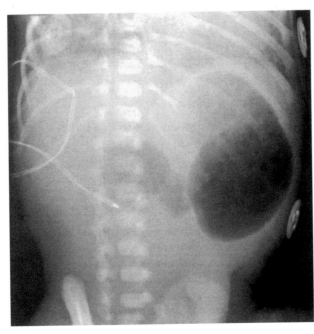

Question 16. (Used with permission of Cedars-Sinai Medical Center, Los Angeles, California.)

17. What syndrome is most associated with the condition in question 16?

A. Turner's syndrome

B. Down syndrome

C. Cri-du-chat syndrome

D. Fragile X syndrome

E. Edward's syndrome

18. A 33-year-old man presents with abdominal pain, nausea, and vomiting. His blood alcohol level is elevated. A KUB is obtained and shows an ileus and sentinel loop in the left upper quadrant. What is the most likely diagnosis?

A. Diverticulitis

B. High-grade small bowel obstruction

C. Sigmoid volvulus

D. Acute pancreatitis

E. Crohn's disease

19. A 64-year-old woman presents to your office with complaints of joint pain and stiffness in the hands and wrists. You notice mild arthritis of bilateral MCP joints and order plain radiographs of the hands and wrists. The films reveal multiple bilateral periarticular joint erosions. What is the most likely diagnosis?

A. Gout

B. Pseudogout

C. Chronic osteomyelitis

D. Rheumatoid arthritis

E. Osteoarthritis

20. A 75-year-old woman who is on chronic warfarin therapy for atrial fibrillation presents to the emergency department after falling from a stepladder. She complains of dizziness and headache. She denies loss of consciousness. A head CT is obtained (Figure Q-20). What is the diagnosis?

A. Epidural hematoma

B. Subdural hematoma

C. Subarachnoid hemorrhage

D. Lymphoma

E. Metastatic lesion

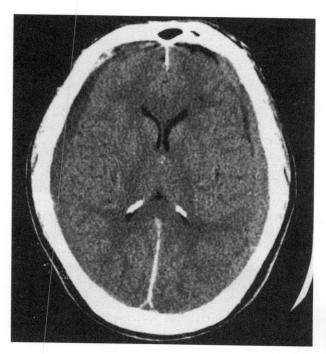

Question 20. (Used with permission of Cedars-Sinai Medical Center, Los Angeles, California.)

21. A 2-year-old child is brought to the emergency department by her mother because the child became tachypneic suddenly while eating. On exam, the child is restless, grunting, and using accessory muscles to breathe. Respiratory rate is 40/min. Temperature is 37.1C. What findings are expected on the chest x-ray?

A. Hyperinflated right lung

B. Alveolar opacification in a lobar distribution

C. Large, spiculated mass

D. Blunting of the costophrenic angle on one side

E. No abnormal findings

22. A 33-year-old man presents to the emergency department with right-sided back pain that radiates to the right groin. The pain began two hours ago and is relatively constant in intensity. Microscopic

hematuria is found on laboratory exam. What is the most appropriate imaging test at this time?

A. Ultrasound

B. Intravenous pyelogram

C. CT urogram

D. KUB

E. MRI of the abdomen

23. A 60-year-old man presents to your office with a chief complaint of left facial swelling and progressive left-sided facial droop for the past three months. You order an imaging study, which is shown below (Figure Q-23). What is the most likely diagnosis?

A. Mumps

B. Parotid carcinoma

C. Stroke

D. Parapharyngeal abscess

E. Pleomorphic adenoma

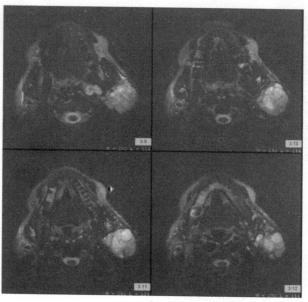

Question 23. (Used with permission of Cedars-Sinai Medical Center, Los Angeles, California.)

24. A 59-year-old man presents to your office complaining of left-sided weakness and recurrent headaches for the past month. You order a CT scan

of the head, which is shown below (Figure Q-24). What is the most likely diagnosis?

A.   Abscesses

B.   Intracerebral hematomas

C.   Multiple Sclerosis

D.   Metastases

E.   Glioblastoma multiforme

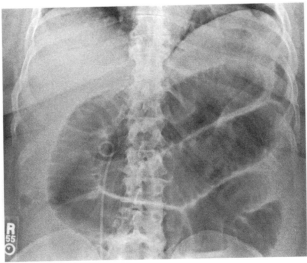

Question 25a. (Used with permission of Cedars-Sinai Medical Center, Los Angeles, California.)

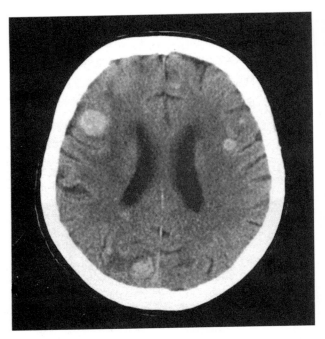

Question 24. (Used with permission of Cedars-Sinai Medical Center, Los Angeles, California.)

25. A 63-year-old woman with a history of ovarian cancer presents to the emergency department with abdominal pain and nausea. Supine and upright abdominal films are shown below (Figures Q-25a, b). What is the most likely diagnosis?

A.   Paralytic ileus

B.   Small bowel obstruction

C.   Colonic obstruction

D.   Pancreatitis with sentinel loop

E.   Fecal impaction

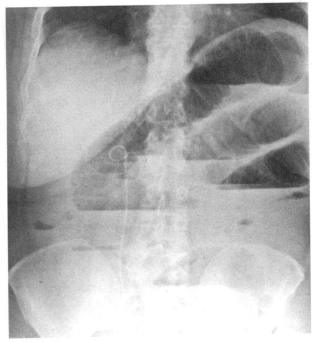

Question 25b. (Used with permission of Cedars-Sinai Medical Center, Los Angeles, California.)

Answers

1. C (Chapter 4)

The PA and lateral chest radiographs are the most useful screening tests in suspected thoracic disease. In this case, the diagnosis is most likely lung cancer, which most likely will be detected by the PA and lateral radiographs. While the chest CT may be useful in staging, it is not an effective screening tool. Sputum cultures would be more useful if the patient had fevers or chills. Bronchoscopy is invasive and not indicated. Chest MRI is not useful in suspected lung parenchymal disease. It is very useful in looking at the heart and mediastinum.

2. B (Chapter 3)

The most appropriate diagnostic test in head trauma with altered level of consciousness is a non-contrast CT scan of the head. Epidural and subdural hematomas are life-threatening and can easily be excluded by non-contrast head CT. A contrast-enhanced head CT is not indicated in trauma as the contrast can mask hemorrhage. Diagnosis of pelvic injury is secondary to intracranial injury. Cervical spine series is indicated, especially if the patient has neck pain; however the patient can be stabilized in a neck collar until after the head CT.

3. D (Chapter 2)

In adults with recurrent sinus infections and/or otitis media, there is an increased incidence of a mass causing an obstruction to the normal drainage from the sinuses and nasal passages. A CT scan of the neck will show the anatomy and rule out any head and neck mass. Skull radiographs are an acceptable screening test for sinusitis but are not useful for excluding head and neck masses.

4. D (Chapter 3)

Hypoattenuation in a vascular distribution is the hallmark of stroke. Combined with the clinical presentation the man likely had a right middle cerebral artery stroke. Hypertension may cause similar symptoms, but radiographically presents as an intraparenchymal hemorrhage, most often in the basal ganglia. Meningitis is not detectable by non-contrast CT; although this could show secondary signs such as hydrocephalus. Carotid artery dissection could present in this way, but is less common. Astrocytoma would appear as a soft tissue mass, surrounded by a ring of low-attenuation edema.

5. B (Chapter 5)

The ultrasound reveals a dilated appendix containing a calcified appendicolith at its proximal end. In children, ultrasound is the preferred test for the diagnosis of appendicitis, due to the lack of ionizing radiation.

6. B (Chapter 7)

Although the Beta-HCG is positive, a normal intrauterine pregnancy is not guaranteed. An ectopic pregnancy may be the cause of the abdominal pain. A CT scan is contraindicated due to the potentially harmful effects of ionizing radiation to the fetus.

---

7.   D (Chapter 5)

Pericholecystic fluid, gallbladder wall thickening, and gallbladder distension are findings associated with (though not diagnostic of) acute cholecystitis.

---

8.   B (Chapter 5)

The CT section through the upper abdomen reveals calcifications within the pancreas and inflammation of the peripancreatic mesenteric fat. Pancreatitis classically presents as upper abdominal pain that radiates through to the back; however, some patients may describe it as chest pain.

---

9.   B (Chapter 9)

The clinical presentation is of croup which is associated with the steeple sign, or a tapering of the trachea on the frontal chest radiograph.

---

10.   C (Chapter 8)

The radiograph of the wrist reveals a torus fracture of the radial metaphysis. This is associated with a fall onto an outstretched hand in a child 5 to 10 years old. A two-month-old would have a bowing type deformity after trauma. A 2-year-old would most likely have a greenstick type fracture. An adult would likely have a Colle's type fracture.

---

11.   B (Chapter 4)

A V/Q scan is the least invasive test that will give the most diagnostic information.

---

12.   D (Chapter 4)

Blunting of the costophrenic angle is a sign of pleural fluid. Following a penetrating wound to the chest, the fluid is most likely blood.

---

13.   C (Chapter 6)

The diagnosis is nephrolithiasis. The patient's history of Crohn's disease is a predisposing factor for developing renal calculi and the microscopic hematuria distinguishes the pain from a gastrointestinal etiology. An intravenous pyelogram could also establish the diagnosis, but in the emergency room situation the non-contrast CT scan is the more appropriate test, due to the decreased radiation exposure and lack of risk from administration of intravenous iodine contrast.

---

14.   B (Chapter 7)

An ultrasound will reveal uterine leiomyomas as hypoechoic areas, which may be mucosal, subserosal, or serosal. An MRI will also provide diagnostic information, but is generally not used as a screening test, but rather if there are remaining diagnostic questions after ultrasound.

---

15.   D (Chapter 4)

Hyperinflation of the lungs and peribronchial inflammation are nonspecific radiologic findings associated with childhood asthma.

---

16.   B (Chapter 9)

The radiograph reveals a "double-bubble" sign, with two large air bubbles in the upper abdomen. These air bubbles represent air in the stomach and duodenal bulb.

---

17.   B (Chapter 9)

Duodenal atresia is associated with Down syndrome. Approximately 30% of babies with duodenal atresia will have Down syndrome. There are also associations with gut malrotation and imperforate anus.

---

18.   D (Chapter 5)

Sentinel loop of bowel is a sign of localized inflammation and is associated with pancreatitis if it is found in the upper abdomen. The elevated alcohol level supports the diagnosis.

19. D (Chapter 8)

Ulnar deviation of the phalanges is classically associated with rheumatoid arthritis. The periarticular erosions may be seen in other conditions such as gout, but this is not the best answer given the rest of the information in the history.

20. B (Chapter 3)

The CT scan of the head shows a new high-attenuation left-sided subdural hematoma. It has the classic biconcave or crescent shape as opposed to an epidural, which has a biconvex, or lens shape. There is also a chronic right-sided subdural hematoma, or hygroma as it is also called when the blood products are replaced by cerebrospinal fluid. A subarachnoid hemorrhage would have high attenuation blood outlining the gyri or in the ventricles. Lymphoma and metastases appear as a mass or multiple masses in the brain parenchyma.

21. A (Chapter 9)

The most likely diagnosis from the history is a foreign body aspiration, from a small piece of food. Most commonly, the food is a pea, a piece of corn, or a small nut. The right lung is more commonly affected, likely because the right mainstem bronchus comes off from the carina at a less acute angle than the left. Hyperinflation is the classic radiographic finding on chest x-ray as the obstruction causes air trapping in the affected lung. Decubitus films will help to prove the diagnosis as the lung with the obstruction remains fully inflated even when it is the dependent side on the decubitus film.

22. C (Chapter 6)

The history is suspicious for a ureteral stone. In the acute setting, a non-contrast CT of the abdomen and pelvis (CT urogram) is the best test for diagnosing a ureteral calculus. An ultrasound may show secondary signs of ureteral obstruction such as dilatation of the renal collecting system and proximal ureter, but is not a good test for locating a ureteral stone. The intravenous pyelogram historically was the test of choice for the diagnosis of ureteral stones, but has been replaced by the CT urogram, which is faster to perform and avoids the use of iodine-based IV contrast. A KUB may show calcifications, but is not a specific test as pelvic phleboliths are common in many patients as well and may interfere with the diagnosis of a distal ureteral stone. MRI of the abdomen is useful for complicated renal masses, some of which may cause hematuria, but is not used for suspected urolithiasis.

23. B (Chapter 2)

The history is consistent with a mass in the parotid gland, which narrows the differential to parotid carcinoma or pleomorphic adenoma. The additional history of facial droop indicates invasion into the seventh cranial nerve, which only a malignant neoplasm would do. Therefore, pleomorphic adenoma is excluded, leaving parotid carcinoma.

Mumps viral infection is uncommon because of vaccinations, would likely be associated with fever and malaise, and would not last for three months. A stroke would not have a facial mass, but might present with a facial droop. A parapharyngeal abscess would also present more acutely and would have a different appearance with a fluid collection in the more medially located parapharyngeal space.

24. D (Chapter 3)

The CT scan reveals multiple round, well-demarcated foci consistent with multiple metastases. Abscesses are not consistent with the history. Intracerebral hematomas would not appear so focal and well circumscribed. Multiple sclerosis does not usually have any findings on CT and can be seen only on MRI. Glioblastoma multiforme is commonly a large infiltrating lesion with surrounding edema.

25. B (Chapter 5)

The radiographs demonstrate a classic appearance of small bowel obstruction with dilated loops of small bowel on the supine film and air-fluid levels on the upright film.

Index

Note: Page numbers followed by f indicate figures; those followed by t indicate tables.

A

Abdominal adhesions, 55, 56f–57f, 59f
Abdominal imaging, 55–69
  of appendicitis, 64–66, 64f–66f
  of Crohn's disease, 58–60, 60f, 61f
  of diverticulitis, 66–69, 67f–69f
  of pancreatitis, 61–63, 62f, 63f
  of small bowel obstruction, 55–58,
    56f–57f, 59f
Abdominal plain film, 58
ACA (anterior cerebral artery), 26
Acoustic schwannoma, 13–16, 13f–17f
Adenocarcinoma, of lung, 38–39,
  41f–43f
Adhesions, abdominal, 55, 56f–57f, 59f
Adnexal mass, 76–78, 76f, 77f
Adnexal structures, 76, 76f
Air bronchograms, 34
"Airspace" pattern, 31
Airway obstruction
  due to foreign body aspiration,
    98–99, 99f–101f
  due to meconium aspiration,
    108–110, 109f
Alveolar pattern, 31
Angiography, magnetic resonance, 22
Ankle, Salter-Harris II fracture of,
  91f–92f
Anterior cerebral artery (ACA), 26
Anterior-posterior (AP) projection,
  31, 33f

Appendicitis, 64–66, 64f–66f
Appendicolith, 66, 66f
Arteriovenous malformation,
    intracerebral hematoma due to,
    26, 27f
Arthritis, rheumatoid, 94–97, 96f
Aspiration
  foreign body, 98–99, 99f–101f
  meconium, 108–110, 109f
Asthma, 38, 39f–40f
Attenuation
  in computed tomography, 3
  in radiography, 1–2

B

Bell-clapper deformity, 73, 73f
"Blowout fractures," of orbital floor, 9
Bone growth plate, 89, 89f
Bone scan, 5
Brain tumor, hemorrhage due to,
  26, 28f
Bronchial obstruction
  due to foreign body aspiration,
    98–99, 99f–101f
  due to meconium aspiration,
    108–110, 109f
Bronchoalveolar carcinoma,
  38–39, 40
Bronchogenic carcinoma, 38–40,
  41f–43f
Bronchograms, air, 34

Bronchopneumonia, 35–38, 37f
"Buckle" fracture, 86, 88f

C

Calculi, renal, 70–71, 70f, 72f–73f
Calvarium, fractures of, 9
Cancer
  head and neck, 16–21, 18f–20f
  lung, 38–40, 41f–43f
Carcinoma
  bronchogenic, 38–40, 41f–43f
  endometrial, 80–82, 81f–82f
  ovarian, 78–80, 79f, 79t
  parotid, 19f, 21
  pterygopalatine fossa, 20f, 21
Cardiac silhouette, 44
Cardiomegaly, 43–45, 48f, 49f
Cerebral arteries, 26, 29f, 30f
Chest radiograph, 31, 32f–33f
Children, 98–110
  duodenal stenosis in,
    103–108, 107f–108f, 109
  foreign body aspiration in, 98–99,
    99f–101f
  meconium aspiration in, 108–110,
    109f
  respiratory distress syndrome in,
    99–103, 102f–106f, 106
Colic, renal, 71
Colles' fracture, 83–86, 83f–85f
"Colon cutoff sign," 62–63

Colonic diverticula, 66–69, 67f–69f
Computed tomography (CT),
    3–4, 4f, 4t
  of endometrial carcinoma, 81,
    81f–82f
  of head and neck, 8, 9
  of intracranial pathology, 22–23
  of small bowel obstruction, 58, 59f
Computed tomography (CT)
    urogram, 71, 73f
Contrast material, 7
Contrecoup injury, 26
Cortical contusion, 26
Coup injury, 24–26
Crohn's disease, 58–60, 60f, 61f
CT. *See* Computed tomography (CT)
Cuffing, peribronchial, 38, 39f, 40f
Cullen's sign, 62
Cyst(s), adnexal dermoid, 76, 76f

D
Dermoid cyst, adnexal, 76, 76f
Diaphysis, 89, 89f
Diethylene triamine penta-acetic acid
    (DTPA) renal scan, 5
Diffusion-weighted imaging (DWI),
    30, 30f
Di-isopropyl iminodiacetic acid
    (DISIDA) scan, 5
Diverticulitis, 66–69, 67f–69f
"Double-bubble" sign, 107, 107f
Duodenal stenosis, 103–108,
    107f–108f, 109
Duodenum, 55

E
Echogenicity, 6
Edema
  peribronchial, 38, 39f, 40f
  pulmonary, 45–53, 50f
Effusion
  pleural, 51f–53f, 53–54
  subpulmonic, 54
Endometrial carcinoma, 80–82,
    81f–82f
Endometrial echo complex (EEC),
    80, 82
Endometrial stripe, 80, 82
Epididymo-orchitis, 75
Epidural hematoma, 23–24, 23f
Epiphysis, 89, 89f
Extra-axial pathology, 22
Extradural lesions, 22

F
Facial bone fractures, 8–9, 9f–12f
Female reproductive organs, normal
    anatomy of, 76, 76f
Femoral fractures, 90–94, 94f, 95f
Fimbriae, 76, 76f
Fluoroscopy, 1–3, 1f
Forearm
  Colles' fracture of, 83–86, 83f–85f
  Smith fracture of, 86, 87f
Foreign body aspiration, 98–99,
    99f–101f
Fracture(s)
  of calvarium, 9
  Colles', 83–86, 83f–85f
  epiphyseal, 90, 90f–93f
  facial bone, 8–9, 9f–12f
  greenstick, 89, 89f
  hip (femoral), 90–94, 94f, 95f
  intertrochanteric, 95f
  occult, 94
  orbital, 9, 9f, 10f
  radiographic description of, 83
  Salter-Harris, 89–90, 89f–93f
  sinus, 9, 11f
  skull-base, 9, 12f
  Smith, 86, 87f
  subcapital, 94
  subtrochanteric, 90
  torus ("buckle"), 86, 88f

G
Gallium scan, 5
Gallstones, 63
Gamma camera, 5, 5f
Glasgow coma scale (GCS), 26
Greenstick fractures, 89, 89f
Grey Turner's sign, 62
Growth plate, 89, 89f
Gynecologic imaging, 76–82
  anatomic basis for, 76, 76f
  of endometrial carcinoma, 80–82,
    81f–82f
  of ovarian carcinoma, 78–80,
    79f, 79t
  of ovarian torsion, 76–78,
    76f–78f, 77t

H
Haustra, 55
Head, 8–21
  acoustic (vestibulocochlear)
    schwannoma of, 13–16, 13f–17f

cancer of, 16–21, 18f–20f
  trauma to, 8–9, 9f–12f, 23–30
Hematoma
  epidural, 23–24, 23f
  intracerebral, 24–26, 27f, 28f
  subdural, 24, 25f
Hemorrhage, intraparenchymal,
    24–26, 27f, 28f
Hernia, incarcerated inguinal, 75
Hilar lymph node enlargement,
    in sarcoidosis, 42, 46f–47f
Hip fracture, 90–94, 94f, 95f
Hounsfield units (HU), 3, 4t
Hyaline membrane disease, 99–103,
    102f–106f, 106
Hydronephrosis, 71

I
Ileum, 55
Ileus, paralytic, 62
Indium tagged white blood cell scan, 5
Infection, pulmonary, 34–38,
    35f–37f
Inguinal hernia, incarcerated, 75
Interfaces, on radiography, 2–3,
    2f–3f
Internal auditory canals, 13,
    13f, 14f
Intertrochanteric fracture, 95f
Intra-axial pathology, 22
Intracerebral hematoma, 24–26,
    27f, 28f
Intracranial pathology, 22
Intradural lesions, 22
Intramedullary lesions, 22
Intraparenchymal hemorrhage, 24–26,
    27f, 28f
Intravenous iodine-based contrast, 7
Intravenous pyelogram (IVP), 71
Iodine-123 scan, 5
Iodine-based contrast, 7

J
Jejunum, 55

K
Kidneys, ureters, and bladder
    radiograph (KUB)
  of nephrolithiasis, 71, 72f
  of small bowel obstruction,
    55, 56f–57f, 58
Kidney stones, 70–71, 70f,
    72f–73f

L

Lace-like pattern, 31
Large cell carcinoma, of lung, 39
Lateral projection, 31, 32f
Level, in computed tomography, 4
Lobar pneumonia, 34, 35f–36f
Lung(s)
    on chest radiograph, 31
    metastases to, 40–42, 44f–45f
Lung cancer, 38–40, 41f–43f
Lung neoplasm, 38–42, 41f–45f
Lung nodule, 38–42, 41f–45f
Lymphadenopathy, in sarcoidosis,
    42, 46f–47f

M

Magnetic resonance (MR)
        angiography, 22
Magnetic resonance imaging (MRI),
        6–7, 6f
    of intracranial pathology, 22, 23
Mastoid cells, fluid in, 9, 12f
Maxillary sinus fractures, 9, 11f
MCA (middle cerebral artery), 26, 29f
McBurney's point, 64
Meconium aspiration, 108–110, 109f
Mediastinum, on chest radiograph, 33
Metaphysis, 89, 89f
Metastases, pulmonary, 40–42, 44f–45f
Middle cerebral artery (MCA), 26, 29f
MR (magnetic resonance)
        angiography, 22
MRI (magnetic resonance imaging),
        6–7, 6f
    of intracranial pathology, 22, 23
Musculoskeletal imaging, 83–97
    of Colles' fracture, 83–86, 83f–85f
    of hip fracture, 90–94, 94f, 95f
    of rheumatoid arthritis, 94–97, 96f
    of Salter-Harris fracture, 89–90,
        89f–93f
    of Smith fracture, 86, 87f
    of torus fracture, 86, 88f

N

Neck cancer, 16–21, 18f–20f
Neoplasm. *See also* Cancer; Carcinoma
    lung, 38–42, 41f–45f
Nephrolithiasis, 70–71, 70f, 72f–73f
Neurofibromatosis (NF), 13
Neurologic imaging, 22–30
    anatomy and general principles of,
        22–23

of epidural hematoma, 23–24, 23f
    for head trauma, 23–30
    of intracerebral hematoma, 24–26,
        27f, 28f
    of stroke, 26–30, 29f, 30f
    of subdural hematoma, 24, 25f
Newborn, transient tachypnea of the,
        103, 104f
NF (neurofibromatosis), 13
Nodule(s), lung, 38–42, 41f–45f
Nuclear medicine, 5, 5f

O

Obstipation, 55
Obstruction
    airway
        due to foreign body aspiration,
            98–99, 99f–101f
        due to meconium aspiration,
            108–110, 109f
    small bowel, 55–58, 56f–57f, 59f
Obturator sign, 65
Occult fractures, 94
Orbital fractures, 9, 9f, 10f
Ovarian carcinoma, 78–80, 79f, 79t
Ovarian mass, 77f
Ovarian torsion, 76–78, 76f–78f, 77t

P

Pancreatitis, 61–63, 62f, 63f
PA (posterior-anterior) projection,
        31, 32f
Paralytic ileus, 62
Paranasal sinuses, fractures of,
        8, 9, 11f
Parotid carcinoma, 19f, 21
Parotid glands, 18f
PCAs (posterior cerebral arteries),
        26, 30f
Pediatric imaging, 98–110
    of duodenal stenosis, 103–108,
        107f–108f, 109
    of foreign body aspiration, 98–99,
        99f–101f
    of meconium aspiration,
        108–110, 109f
    of respiratory distress syndrome,
        99–103, 102f–106f, 106
Periarticular erosions, 96f, 97
Peribronchial cuffing, 38, 39f, 40f
Peribronchial edema, 38, 39f, 40f
PET (positron emission tomography), 5
Physis, 89, 89f

Pleural effusion, 51f–53f, 53–54
Pneumomediastinum, 103, 106f
Pneumonia
    broncho-, 35–38, 37f
    lobar, 34, 35f–36f
Pneumothorax, 103, 105f
Positron emission tomography
        (PET), 5
Posterior-anterior (PA) projection,
        31, 32f
Posterior cerebral arteries (PCAs),
        26, 30f
Psoas sign, 64–65
Pterygoid plates, 18f
Pterygopalatine fossa carcinoma,
        20f, 21
Pulmonary edema, 45–53, 50f
Pulmonary metastases, 40–42, 44f–45f
Pulmonary nodule, 38–42, 41f–45f
Pulmonary vessels, on chest
        radiograph, 31

R

Radiodensities, 2, 2t
Radiography, 1–3, 1f–3f
    chest, 31, 32f–33f
    kidneys, ureters, and bladder (KUB)
        of nephrolithiasis, 71, 72f
        of small bowel obstruction, 55,
            56f–57f, 58
Radiology, general principles in, 1–7
Radiolucency, 2
Radionuclide, 5
Radius
    Colles' fracture of, 83–86, 83f–85f
    Salter-Harris IV fracture of, 93f
    Smith fracture of, 86, 87f
    torus fracture of, 86, 88f
Renal calculi, 70–71, 70f, 72f–73f
Renal colic, 71
Respiratory distress syndrome (RDS),
        99–103, 102f–106f, 106
"Reticular" pattern, 31
Rheumatoid arthritis, 94–97, 96f
Rheumatoid factor (RF), 94
Roentgen, Wilhelm, 1
"Rose thorn" ulcers, 60, 61f

S

"Sail sign," 106f
Salivary gland tumors, 19f, 21
Salter-Harris fracture, 89–90, 89f–93f
Sarcoidosis, 42–43, 46f–47f

Schwannoma, acoustic
    (vestibulocochlear), 13–16,
    13f–17f
"Sentinel loop," of small bowel, 62
Sinus fractures, 8, 9, 11f
Skip lesions, 58, 60
Skull-base fracture, 9, 12f
Small bowel
    obstruction of, 55–58, 56f–57f, 59f
    "sentinel loop" of, 62
Small cell carcinoma, of lung, 39
Smith fracture, 86, 87f
Sonography. *See* Ultrasonography (US)
Spinal canal lesions, 22
Squamous cell carcinoma, of lung, 39
Stroke, 26–30, 29f, 30f
Subcapital fractures, 94
Subdural hematoma, 24, 25f
Subpulmonic effusion, 54
Subtrochanteric fractures, 90
Swan-neck deformity, 94, 96f

T
Tachypnea, transient, of the newborn,
    103, 104f
Technetium tagged red blood cell
    scan, 5
Testicular torsion, 71–75, 73f, 74f
Thoracic imaging, 31–54
    anatomy and general principles of,
        31–34, 32f–33f
    of asthma, 38, 39f–40f

of bronchogenic carcinoma, 38–40,
    41f–43f
of bronchopneumonia, 35–38, 37f
of cardiomegaly, 43–45, 48f, 49f
of infection, 34–38, 35f–37f
of lobar pneumonia, 34, 35f–36f
of metastases, 40–42, 44f–45f
of neoplasm, 38–42, 41f–45f
of pleural effusion, 51f–53f, 53–54
of pulmonary edema, 45–53, 50f
of sarcoidosis, 42–43, 46f–47f
"Through-transmission," 6
Tibia, torus fracture of, 86
Torsion
    ovarian, 76–78, 76f–78f, 77t
    testicular, 71–75, 73f, 74f
Torus fracture, 86, 88f
Transient tachypnea of the newborn,
    103, 104f
Transvaginal ultrasound
    of endometrial carcinoma,
        80–81, 81f
    of ovarian carcinoma, 79, 79f, 79t
Trauma
    to facial bones, 8–9, 9f–12f
    head, 8–9, 9f–12f, 23–30

U
Ulcers, "rose thorn," 60, 61f
Ultrasonography (US), 5–6, 5f
    of endometrial carcinoma,
        80–81, 81f

of nephrolithiasis, 71
of ovarian carcinoma, 79, 79f, 79t
of testicular torsion, 74–75, 74f
Ureteropelvic junction (UPJ),
    70, 70f
Ureterovesicular junction (UVJ),
    70, 70f
Urogram, CT, 71, 73f
Urolithiasis, 70–71, 70f, 72f–73f
Urologic imaging, 70–75
    of nephrolithiasis, 70–71, 70f,
        72f–73f
    of testicular torsion, 71–75,
        73f, 74f
US. *See* Ultrasonography (US)
UVJ (ureterovesicular junction),
    70, 70f

V
Valvulae conniventes, 55
Vascular malformation, intracerebral
    hematoma due to, 26, 27f
Ventilation/perfusion (V/Q) scan, 5
Vestibulocochlear schwannoma,
    13–16, 13f–17f

W
Window, in computed tomography, 4

X
X-ray(s), 1
X-ray machine, 1, 1f